Medical Management of Insulin-Dependent (Type I) Diabetes

Second Edition

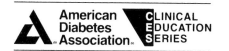

Chief Scientific and Medical Officer
Richard Kahn, PhD

Publisher
Susan H. Lau

Editorial Director
Peter Banks

Managing Editor
Christine B. Welch

Associate Editor
Sherrye Landrum

Director of Production
Carolyn R. Segree

American Diabetes Association, Inc., Alexandria, VA 22314
First printing June 1994
Printed in the United States of America
ISBN 0-945448-36-8

Contents

A Word About This Guide

The *Medical Management of Insulin-Dependent (Type I) Diabetes* is the most recent addition to the American Diabetes Association's Clinical Education Series, which also includes *Medical Management of Non-Insulin-Dependent (Type II) Diabetes*, *Therapy for Diabetes Mellitus and Related Disorders*, and *Medical Management of Pregnancy Complicated by Diabetes*. The Clinical Education Series was designed to provide health-care professionals with the comprehensive information needed to provide the best possible medical care to patients with diabetes mellitus.

This book evolved from the *Physician's Guide to Insulin-Dependent (Type I) Diabetes: Diagnosis and Treatment*. During the last decade, much new information has advanced our knowledge of the natural history and pathogenesis of diabetes and its complications. The results of the Diabetes Control and Complications Trial and other important clinical studies have major implications for the management of type I diabetes. In 1994, the American Diabetes Association completed updated position statements on *Standards of Medical Care for Patients With Diabetes Mellitus* and *Nutrition Recommendations and Principles for People With Diabetes Mellitus* as well as several major technical reviews. From these have emerged key clinical practice recommendations that have been incorporated into this text.

Seventy-two years after the first use of insulin, it is clear that blood glucose regulation, proper nutrition, regular exercise, attention to blood pressure and blood lipid levels, and smoking cessation are key elements in the management of type I diabetes. The development of *Medical Management of Insulin-Dependent (Type I) Diabetes* was designed to provide state-of-the-art information on these issues. Its publication could not have been possible without the expert guidance of the many contributors to the first and present editions. The book's focus on pathogenesis, diagnosis and classification, patient education and self-management training, and maintenance of wellness through proper nutrition, exercise, and the prevention and treatment of complications was the work of many experts. We are particularly indebted to the editor-in-chief of the first edition, Mark A. Sperling, MD, and the many contributors who laid the foundation of the current edition.

With the American Diabetes Association, I trust that you will find this book as useful as its predecessor. Hopefully, it will encourage you to add other American Diabetes Association publications to your library, which can help you manage your patients with diabetes more effectively.

JULIO V. SANTIAGO, MD
Editor-in-Chief

Contributors

Editor-in-Chief   JULIO V. SANTIAGO, MD
St. Louis Children's Hospital
St. Louis, Missouri

Contributing   DAVID E. GOLDSTEIN, MD
Editors   University of Missouri Medical Center
Columbia, Missouri

MOREY HAYMOND, MD
Nemours Children's Clinic
Jacksonville, Florida

JOAN HEINS, MA, RD, CDE
Washington University School of Medicine
St. Louis, Missouri

ALICIA SCHIFFRIN, MD
Montreal Children's Hospital
Montreal, Quebec, Canada

DONALD C. SIMONSON, MD
Joslin Diabetes Center
Boston, Massachusetts

BRUCE R. ZIMMERMAN, MD
Mayo Clinic
Rochester, Minnesota

Reviewers

GEORGE BLANKENSHIP, MD
Pennsylvania State University
Hershey, Pennsylvania

STUART BRINK, MD
New England Diabetes Endocrinology Center
Chestnut Hill, Massachusetts

WILLIAM L. CLARKE, MD
University of Virginia Health Sciences Center
Charlottesville, Virginia

JOHN A. COLWELL, MD, PhD
Medical University of South Carolina
Charleston, South Carolina

ANNE DALY, MS, RD, CDE
Springfield Diabetes and Endocrine Center
Springfield, Illinois

RALPH A. DeFRONZO, MD
University of Texas Health Sciences Center
San Antonio, Texas

JOHN T. DEVLIN, MD
Maine Medical Center
Portland, Maine

JEFFREY B. HALTER, MD
University of Michigan
Ann Arbor, Michigan

FRANCINE KAUFMAN, MD
Children's Hospital of Los Angeles
Los Angeles, California

WILLIAM F. KEANE, MD
Hennepin County Medical Center
Minneapolis, Minnesota

RONALD KLEIN, MD, MPH
University of Wisconsin Medical School
Madison, Wisconsin

ROBERT A. KREISBERG, MD, FACP
University of Alabama
Birmingham, Alabama

DAVIDA F. KRUGER, MSN, RN, C, CDE
Henry Ford Hospital
Detroit, Michigan

MARK LANDON, MD
Ohio State University
Columbus, Ohio

CAROLYN LEONTOS, MS, RD, CDE
University of Nevada
Las Vegas, Nevada

JOHN I. MALONE, MD
University of South Florida
Tampa, Florida

ROBERT A. RIZZA, MD
Mayo Clinic
Rochester, Minnesota

STEPHEN H. SCHNEIDER, MD
Robert Wood Johnson Medical School
New Brunswick, New Jersey

LINDA SIMINERIO, MS, RN, CDE
University of Pittsburgh Children's Hospital
Pittsburgh, Pennsylvania

JAY S. SKYLER, MD
University of Miami
Miami, Florida

MARK A. SPERLING, MD
University of Pittsburgh Children's Hospital
Pittsburgh, Pennsylvania

SUZANNE STROWIG, MSN, RN, CDE
University of Texas Southwestern Medical Center
Dallas, Texas

Diagnosis and Classification/ Pathogenesis

Highlights

Classification and Diagnosis

Pathogenesis

Highlights
Diagnosis and Classification/
Pathogenesis

CLASSIFICATION AND DIAGNOSIS

Diabetes mellitus is classified into four clinically (and possibly pathogenetically) different types:
- insulin-dependent diabetes (type I or IDDM),
- non-insulin-dependent diabetes (type II or NIDDM),
- secondary diabetes, i.e., diabetes due to or associated with certain diseases of the pancreas, hormonal syndromes, drugs, and rare conditions involving the insulin receptor and other genetic syndromes, and
- malnutrition-related diabetes mellitus, which occurs most in developing countries in young, obviously lean individuals.

Indications for diagnostic testing include
- positive screening test results,
- obvious signs and symptoms of diabetes mellitus (polydipsia, polyuria, polyphagia, weight loss), and
- an incomplete clinical picture, such as glucosuria or equivocal elevation of random plasma glucose level.

When diabetes is fully evolved, fasting plasma glucose levels exceed 140 mg/dl (>7.8 mM), and random plasma glucose levels exceed 200 mg/dl (>11.1 mM).

The incidence of type I diabetes is 15 in 100,000/yr among people <20 yr old, similar in males and females, lower in African Americans than whites, and markedly less common in Hispanics, Asian Americans, and American Indians.

At presentation, patients with type I diabetes are usually <30 yr old, lean, and often have experienced significant weight loss, polyuria, and polydipsia before presentation. The oral glucose tolerance test is rarely needed to

diagnose type I diabetes. Delayed diagnosis is a serious, sometimes fatal problem, especially among younger children.

Approximately 40% of children <2 yr old present in coma and, of these, ~5% die.

Type I diabetes can develop at any age and is sometimes mistaken for type II diabetes among older patients.

PATHOGENESIS

The primary defect in type I diabetes is inadequate insulin secretion by pancreatic β-cells.

Genetic predisposition clearly plays a role in development of type I diabetes. However, environmental factors may be involved in initiating β-cell destruction, which is carried out by an autoimmune process not completely understood.

Detectable abnormalities of insulin secretion may be preceded by months to years of β-cell destruction, noted by the presence of islet cell antibodies.

Fasting hyperglycemia occurs when β-cell mass is reduced by 80–90%. Typical symptoms of diabetes, i.e., polyuria, polydipsia, and weight loss, appear once hyperglycemia exceeds the renal threshold of ~180 mg/dl (~10.0 mM) glucose.

Sometime after diagnosis and correction of acute metabolic abnormalities, some individuals experience a "honeymoon phase," a temporary period when need for exogenous insulin is diminished or absent.

Within 8–10 yr after clinical presentation, β-cell loss is complete; at this point, insulin deficiency is absolute, and circulating islet cell antibodies can no longer be detected.

Diagnosis and Classification

INTRODUCTION

Diabetes mellitus is a chronic disorder that is, *1)* characterized by hyperglycemia, *2)* associated with major abnormalities in carbohydrate, fat, and protein metabolism, and *3)* accompanied by a marked propensity to develop relatively specific forms of renal, ocular, neurologic, and premature cardiovascular diseases. Diabetes encompasses a wide clinical spectrum and is classified into four different types:

■ insulin-dependent (type I) diabetes,
■ non-insulin-dependent (type II) diabetes,
■ secondary diabetes (diabetes mellitus associated with certain conditions and syndromes), and
■ malnutrition-related diabetes mellitus.

Although type I diabetes accounts for ~10% of all diagnosed cases of diabetes, its immediate risks and stringent acute treatment requirements demand rapid recognition, diagnosis, and management.

This chapter explores characteristics that differentiate type I diabetes from other forms of diabetes, discusses criteria for correct diagnosis, and illustrates various clinical presentations.

CRITERIA FOR DIAGNOSIS

Diabetes is diagnosed when the fasting plasma glucose concentration exceeds 140 mg/dl (7.8 mM) and/or random plasma glucose levels exceed 200 mg/dl (11.1 mM) on more than one occasion with or without overt symptoms of diabetes. The clinical signs and/or symptoms that accompany diabetes are polyuria, polydipsia, fatigue, polyphagia, weight loss, or blurred vision and persistent hyperglycemia. In the young child or infant, these signs or symptoms are frequently missed until the child presents with unexplained dehydration, acidosis, and/or a severe candidal diaper rash. Under the above circumstances, an oral glucose tolerance test (OGTT) is not needed, and its use is contraindicated (Table 1.1). In fact, an OGTT is rarely needed to diagnose type I diabetes.

Although not considered diagnostic, an elevated glycated hemoglobin may confirm the presence of significant pre-existing hyperglycemia (barring the presence of a hemoglobin variant). Impaired glucose tolerance, as distinguished from diabetes mellitus, refers to abnormal plasma glucose values that do not meet the established criteria to diagnose diabetes and may or may not be predictive of diabetes. Because the diagnosis of diabetes has profound effects on an individual's ability to obtain affordable health care and life insurance and may affect their vocational careers, great care should be taken in not labeling an individual with impaired glucose tolerance as having diabetes.

RISK OF DEVELOPING TYPE I DIABETES

Although type I diabetes is much less common in the general population than type II diabetes, type I diabetes is by no means rare among children and young adults. There is an estimated annual incidence of 12–14 cases/100,000 people under age 20 yr and a prevalance of 1 case/500 young people under age 16 yr. It is one of the most common childhood diseases: it is three- to fourfold more common than chronic childhood diseases such as cystic fibrosis, juvenile rheumatoid arthritis, or leukemia, and it is nearly tenfold more common than nephrotic syndrome or muscular dystrophy.

The annual incidence decreases after age 20 yr. Incidence is similar in men and women; it is lower in African Americans, Hispanics, Asian Americans, and American Indians than in whites.

The risk of diabetes to family members of an individual with type I diabetes is significantly higher compared to the general population. The statistical risk of a family member developing type I diabetes is linked to the genetic similarities of the family members. For example, when one identical twin develops diabetes, the risk to the other twin is 25–50%. This is in contrast to a 0.4% risk in the general population, a 15% risk

Table 1.1. Diagnosis of Diabetes Mellitus in Nonpregnant Adults

Diagnosis of diabetes mellitus in nonpregnant adults should be restricted to those who have *one* of the following:

■ random plasma glucose level ≥200 mg/dl (≥11.1 mM) *plus* classic signs and symptoms of diabetes mellitus including polydipsia, polyuria, polyphagia, and weight loss, and blurred vision; or

■ fasting plasma glucose level ≥140 mg/dl (≥7.7 mM) on at least 2 occasions; or

■ fasting plasma glucose level <140 mg/dl (<7.7 mM) plus sustained elevated plasma glucose levels during at least 2 oral glucose tolerance tests. The 2-h sample and at least one other between 0 and 2 h after 75-g glucose dose should be ≥200 mg/dl (≥11.1 mM). Oral glucose tolerance testing is not necessary if patient has fasting plasma glucose level of ≥140 mg/dl (≥7.7 mM).*

*An OGTT is rarely needed to diagnose type I diabetes.

in an HLA identical sibling, and a 1% risk in an HLA nonidentical sibling.

DISTINGUISHING TYPE I DIABETES FROM OTHER FORMS

Type I Diabetes

Type I diabetes can develop at any age. Although most cases are diagnosed before the patient is 30 yr old, it also occurs in older individuals. Because patients with type I diabetes are insulinopenic, insulin therapy is essential to prevent rapid and severe dehydration, catabolism, ketoacidosis, and death (Table 1.2). Most patients are lean and have experienced significant weight loss, polyuria, polydipsia, and fatigue before presentation. At presentation, they have significant elevations of glycated hemoglobin, providing evidence of weeks, if not months, of hyperglycemia. In addition, 65–85% have circulating antibodies directed against the islet cells, and 20–60% have antibodies directed against insulin.

Type II Diabetes

In contrast, patients with type II diabetes generally present after age 30, are not prone to develop ketoacidosis unless severely stressed physiologically, are generally but not always obese, may be asymptomatic or only mildly symptomatic, and usually have a family history of diabetes. A form of type II diabetes with childhood onset (maturity-onset diabetes of the young [MODY]) is a well-described but rare autosomal dominant disorder.

Patients with type II diabetes are not absolutely dependent on exogenous insulin for survival, although insulin therapy is often employed to lower blood glucose levels (Table 1.2).

Not Quite Type I or II Diabetes

Some patients are difficult to categorize as having type I or type II diabetes. Currently, there is no routinely available test that reliably differentiates between the two types. Generally, if the patient is <30 yr old, not obese, and has signs and symptoms of diabetes mellitus and an elevated fasting plasma glucose, the physician should assume type I diabetes and treat with insulin. The presence of moderate ketonuria with hyperglycemia in an otherwise unstressed individual strongly supports a diagnosis of type I diabetes, whereas the absence or modest ketonuria is of no diagnostic value.

Clinicians should also be aware that some cases presenting as type II diabetes may subsequently be discovered to be type I diabetes. In these individuals, antibodies to islet cell components may indicate the eventual need for insulin therapy. These patients are usually lean, and their insulin requirements increase as they develop manifestations of complete insulin deficiency. In contrast, adolescents and young adults who present with typical signs and symptoms of type I diabetes later require insulin treatment only intermittently. Table 1.3 illustrates specific conditions often associated with the other forms of diabetes and glucose intolerance. Further studies are required to determine the pathophysiology of these conditions.

Table 1.2. Types of Diabetes Mellitus and Other Categories of Abnormal Glucose Metabolism

CLINICAL CLASSES	DISTINGUISHING CHARACTERISTICS
Diabetes mellitus	
Insulin-dependent diabetes mellitus (IDDM or type II)	Patients may be of any age, are not usually obese, and often have abrupt onset of signs and symptoms with insulinopenia before age 30. These patients often have strongly positive urine ketone tests in conjunction with hyperglycemia and are dependent on insulin therapy to prevent ketoacidosis and to sustain life.
Non-insulin-dependent diabetes mellitus (NIDDM or type II) (obese or nonobese)	Patients usually are >30 yr at diagnosis, obese, and have relatively few classic symptoms. They are not prone to ketoacidosis except during periods of stress. Although not dependent on exogenous insulin for survival, they may require it for adequate control of hyperglycemia.
Secondary and other types of diabetes	Patients with secondary and other types of diabetes mellitus have certain associated conditions or syndromes (see Table 1.3).
Malnutrition-related diabetes mellitus*	Patients are young (between 10 and 40 yr old), usually symptomatic, and not prone to ketoacidosis, but most require insulin therapy.
Impaired glucose tolerance (IGT) (obese or nonobese)	Patients with impaired glucose tolerance have plasma glucose levels that are higher than normal but not diagnostic for diabetes mellitus.
Gestational diabetes mellitus (GDM)	Patients with gestational diabetes mellitus have onset or discovery of glucose intolerance during pregnancy.

*Recommended as a separate clinical class of diabetes mellitus by the World Health Organization (WHO); see Bibliography.
Adapted from classification developed by an international work group sponsored by the National Diabetes Data Group, National Institutes of Health; see Bibliography.

CLINICAL PRESENTATION OF TYPE I DIABETES

The presentation of type I diabetes covers a broad range, from mild nonspecific symptoms or no symptoms to coma. In children, correct diagnosis is often delayed because polyuria is incorrectly attributed to urinary tract infection or enuresis; anorexia rather than polyphagia may occur; and fatigue, irritability, weight loss, deterioration of school performance, and secondary enuresis are ascribed to emotional problems. In some cases, "failure to thrive" may be an overlooked indication of diabetes in a young child.

Fewer patients with previously undiagnosed type I diabetes are presenting in severe diabetic ketoacidosis than in the past, and >70% of cases are diagnosed within 1 mo of onset of symptoms. Nevertheless, delayed diagnosis continues to be a serious and occasionally fatal problem, especially among younger children. The symptoms of polyuria are less obvious in the young child and are frequently missed until metabolic de-

Table 1.3. Secondary Diabetes Mellitus and Impaired Glucose Tolerance

SECONDARY TO:

Pancreatic disease	Examples: pancreatectomy, hemochromatosis, cystic fibrosis, chronic pancreatitis
Endocrinopathies	Examples: Cushing's syndrome, acromegaly, pheochromocytoma, primary aldosteronism, glucagonoma
Drugs and chemical agents	Examples: certain antihypertensive drugs, thiazide diuretics, glucocorticoids, estrogen-containing preparations, nicotinic acid, phenytoin, catecholamines

ASSOCIATED WITH:

Insulin receptor abnormalities	Examples: acanthosis nigricans
Genetic syndromes	Examples: lipodrystophic syndromes, muscular dystrophies, Huntington's chorea
Miscellaneous conditions	Example: polycystic ovary disease

For a more complete list, see National Diabetes Data Group, in Bibliography.

compensation has occurred. These very young children frequently present with severe dehydration, metabolic acidosis, and a clinical history that is inconsistent with the severity of their clinical appearance, e.g., absence of diarrhea or significant vomiting. Because of the delay in the diagnosis of the younger child, the frequency of coma as a presenting feature in children <2 yr of age is considerably greater than those of older children, adolescents, and adults. In young adults, the presentation is often less acute, although an absolute requirement for insulin becomes evident with time.

CONCLUSION

Patients with type I diabetes are dependent on insulin for as long as they live. Any lean individual <30 yr of age with typical signs and symptoms of hyperglycemia should be assumed to have type I diabetes. A high index of suspicion is needed to diagnose diabetes in very young children or elderly patients.

BIBLIOGRAPHY

American Diabetes Association position statement: Office guide to diagnosis and classification of diabetes mellitus and other categories of glucose intolerance. *Diabetes Care* 16 (Suppl. 2): 4, 1993

National Diabetes Data Group: Classification and diagnosis of diabetes mellitus and other categories of glucose intolerance. *Diabetes* 28: 1039–57, 1979

World Health Organization: *Diabetes mellitus: report of a WHO study group.* Geneva, World Health Org., 1985 (Tech. Rep. Ser., no. 727)

Pathogenesis

INTRODUCTION

The primary defect in insulin-dependent (type I) diabetes mellitus is decreased insulin secretion by pancreatic β-cells. This single defect accounts for the hyperglycemia, polyuria, polydipsia, and weight loss, dehydration, electrolyte disturbance, and ketoacidosis observed in patients presenting for the first time with type I diabetes. The capacity of normal pancreatic β-cells to secrete insulin is far in excess of that normally needed to control carbohydrate, fat, and protein metabolism. As a result, clinical onset is preceded by an extensive asymptomatic period during which β-cells are inexorably destroyed. The evolving process of β-cell destruction reaches a point where insufficient insulin is secreted to maintain normal plasma glucose concentrations, which causes the broadly predictable abnormalities in carbohydrate, fat, and protein metabolism characterizing the uncontrolled diabetic condition.

PATHOPHYSIOLOGY OF THE CLINICAL ONSET OF TYPE I DIABETES

Insulin is the primary hormone that suppresses hepatic glucose production, lipolysis, and proteolysis. It increases the transport of glucose into adipocytes and myocytes and stimulates glycogen synthesis. In the presence of adequate plasma amino acids, insulin maintains or perhaps stimulates whole-body protein anabolism. As such, insulin is the primary hormone of anabolism of meal-derived nutrients (Table 1.4).

In the postabsorptive state, the plasma concentration of glucose is maintained in a narrow range (80–95 mg/dl [4.4–5.3 mM]) by precise regulation of hepatic glucose release and peripheral glucose utilization. Basal plasma insulin concentrations maintain hepatic glucose release at a rate of 1.9–2.1 mg · kg^{-1} · min^{-1} (10–12 μM · kg^{-1}· min^{-1}). This is of critical importance to provide adequate glucose for the brain, which accounts for nearly 50% of total glucose utilization under these conditions. With prolonged fasting, the plasma insulin concentration decreases even further, permitting increased mobilization of free fatty acids (FFA). The resulting increase in circulating FFA concentration drives hepatic ketogenesis, which results in ketosis. Increased availability of plasma FFA, β-hydroxybutyrate, and acetoacetate provide alternative metabolic fuels to glucose and reduce the rates of glucose utilization by peripheral tissues and brain.

After ingestion of a mixed meal, nearly 85% of ingested glucose enters the systemic circulation. The increasing arterial glucose concentration stimulates the secretion of insulin into the portal vein. About half of the secreted insulin is extracted by the liver, which signals the suppression of hepatic glucose release. The unextracted insulin enters the systemic circulation, where it stimulates glucose uptake, primarily by muscle, and decreases lipolysis and proteolysis. This facilitates a continuous entry of glucose into the systemic circulation by permitting a switch from endogenous glucose production to exogenous glucose. As dietary glucose entry decreases with the absorption of the meal-derived carbohydrate, plasma glucose decreases as does the secretion and plasma concentration of insulin. When plasma glucose reaches or even falls slightly below basal concentrations, hepatic glucose production is again increased by both the decrease in plasma insulin and by an increase in plasma glucagon concentration (Table 1.4).

PROGRESSION OF METABOLIC ABNORMALITIES DURING ONSET

The insulin secretory reserves of the normal pancreas are considerable. Therefore, individuals destined to develop type I diabetes go through a variable interval of months to years of autoimmune β-cell destruction before abnormalities in insulin secretion or glucose metabolism can be detected (Figure 1.1).

The earliest detectable abnormality in insulin secretion is a progressive

Table 1.4. Physiologic Effects of High- Versus Low-Insulin States

	HIGH-INSULIN (FED) STATE	LOW-INSULIN (FASTED) STATE
Liver	Glucose uptake Glycogen synthesis Lipogenesis Absent ketogenesis Absent gluconeogenesis	Glucose production Glycogenolysis Absent lipogenesis Ketogenesis Gluconeogenesis
Muscle	Glucose uptake Glucose oxidation Glycogen synthesis Sustained protein synthesis	Absent glucose uptake Fatty acid, ketone oxidation Glycogenolysis Proteolysis and amino acid release
Adipose tissue	Glucose uptake Lipid synthesis Triglyceride uptake	Absent glucose uptake Lipolysis and fatty acid release Absent triglyceride uptake

reduction of the immediate (first-phase) plasma insulin response during intravenous glucose tolerance testing. This impairment alone has little deleterious effect on overall glucose homeostasis: fasting plasma glucose concentrations remain normal, and the response to an oral glucose tolerance test is virtually unimpaired. At this stage of the disease, most affected individuals have circulating antibodies to islet cells components, islet cell antibodies (ICAs), or to their own insulin. These are markers of an ongoing autoimmune process that eventuates in type I diabetes. The presence of significant titers of either, or the combination of circulating antibodies to insulin and ICAs, together with impaired first-phase insulin secretion, appear predictive of type I diabetes (Figure 1.1).

CLINICAL ONSET OF DIABETIC SYMPTOMS AND METABOLIC DECOMPENSATION

When ongoing destruction has reduced β-cell mass by 80–90%, the individual's insulin secretory capacity becomes insufficient to regulate normally hepatic glucose production (Figure 1.1). Initially, only postprandial hyperglycemia occurs, reflecting a failure to suppress adequately hepatic glucose production during meal absorption together with some decrease in peripheral glucose utilization. But as insulin secretion is further compromised, progressive fasting hyperglycemia occurs as a result of increased basal hepatic glucose production and decreased glucose uptake by peripheral tissue. Hyperglycemia per se may further compromise glucose utilization by reducing the number and/or activity of glucose transporters available on both insulin-dependent and non-insulin-dependent tissues.

When the plasma glucose concentration exceeds the renal threshold of ~180 mg/dl (10.0 mM), glucosuria results in an osmotic diuresis, generating the classic symptoms of polyuria and a compensatory polydipsia. If untreated, the symptoms usually progress as the hyperglycemia and glucosuria increase. With evolving insulin deficiency, weight loss occurs as body fat and protein stores are reduced due to increased rates of lipolysis and proteolysis. With the superimposed metabolic abnormalities of diabetes itself or with a minor viral or bacterial infection, plasma concentrations of glucagon, growth hormone, epinephrine, and cortisol increase. These hormones antagonize insulin's effect, further promoting hepatic glucose pro-

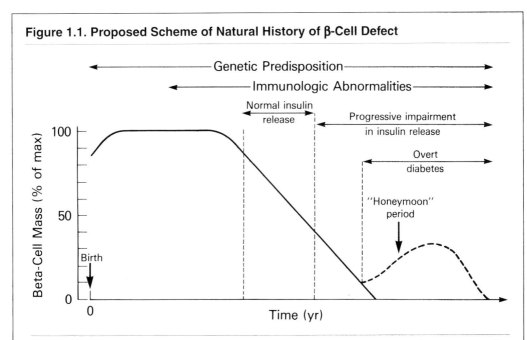

Figure 1.1. Proposed Scheme of Natural History of β-Cell Defect

Timing of trigger in relation to immunologic abnormalities is unknown. Note that overt diabetes is not apparent until insulin secretory reserves are <10–20% of normal.

duction (by stimulating both glycogenolysis and gluconeogenesis), lipolysis, ketogenesis, and proteolysis. As long as fluid intake is sufficient to offset the fluid losses resulting from the combined diuresis of both glucosuria and ketonuria, some individuals can remain compensated for weeks, if not months. Should the individual be unable to consume adequate amounts of fluid as a result of nausea from the ketosis or due to an intercurrent illness, rapid and severe losses of both intra- and extracellular fluid and electrolytes can ensue and, in the course of hours, lead to a clinical presentation of severe ketoacidosis.

Honeymoon Phase

At initial presentation with symptomatic hyperglycemia and/or ketosis, circulating insulin concentrations are low, and there is no significant β-cell response to any of the usual insulin secretagogues. Initially, exogenous insulin require-

ments are relatively large, due not only to the reduced insulin secretion but also to insulin resistance.

After the correction of the hyperglycemia, metabolic acidosis, and ketosis, endogenous insulin secretion recovers (Figure 1.1). During this time, exogenous insulin requirements may decrease dramatically. During the honeymoon period, which may last for up to 1 yr, good metabolic control may be easily achieved. The need for increasing exogenous insulin replacement is inevitable, however, and should always be anticipated. As a result, strict attention to diet and to self-monitoring of blood glucose must be maintained throughout this period to avoid recurrence of ketoacidosis, a life-threatening event.

Finally, within 5 yr for children and 10 yr after clinical presentation regardless of age at presentation, β-cell destruction is essentially complete. At this point, insulin deficiency is absolute.

Immune Therapy

The role of several immune therapies in preserving the remaining β-cells before metabolic decompensation have been studied in individuals at the clinical onset of diabetes (prolonged, asymptomatic phase). Early therapeutic attempts centered mainly on general immune suppression. Although effective in prolonging the honeymoon period, none resulted in permanent remission. The risk(s) of such therapies make them unacceptable for clinical use. Newer approaches seek to resume a state of immune tolerance to islet cells and/or to abrogate immune effects (e.g., free radical generation) in individuals with prediabetes.

These intervention trials offer an opportunity to preserve a significant mass of β-cells and potentially prevent or delay overt diabetes. Potential therapeutic modalities must be approached with caution and should be utilized only in conjunction with a multicenter scientific study.

GENETICS AND IMMUNOLOGY OF TYPE I DIABETES

Type I diabetes is a genetically influenced and immunologically mediated disease with a prolonged asymptomatic phase (prediabetes), which results in progressive β-cell destruction, insulin deficiency, and overt clinical symptoms. The identity of the initiating event(s) remains speculative. Predisposition to type I diabetes is inherited as a heterogeneous, multigenic trait with low penetrance and gender biases, which has created major obstacles to the identification of the "diabetes gene(s)." However, it is known that diabetes occurs in multiple family members of a person with type I diabetes in ~15% of cases and is more common among identical twins (25–50%) than fraternal twins (6%) (Table 1.5).

An association exists between type I diabetes and the class I human leukocyte antigens (HLA) B8 and B15. An even closer association exists with the HLA class II DR3 and DR4 molecules. These molecules (DR3, DR4, DQ) are comprised of an α- and a β-chain, which present processed antigen to T lymphocytes. In the presentation of the processed antigen, the class II DQ molecules appear to be more closely associated with type I diabetes, whereas other molecules decreased the risk (DR2). Of particular importance in the presentation of a processed antigen is the identity of the amino acid at position 57 of the DQ β-chain. This critical residue may maintain the structural conformation of the DQ antigen-binding cleft. A neutral amino acid (valine, alanine, serine) in position 57 (non-asp) confers a higher risk of type I diabetes than that transmitted by alleles containing a charged aspartic acid residue (asp-positive). The variability of type I diabetes prevalence throughout the world tends to correlate positively with the frequency of the DQ alleles (DQ non-asp) in the geographic populations studied.

Although the DQ-β aspartate-57 hypothesis is attractive, this model may be oversimplified. In addition, sex-linked biases of diabetes susceptibility genes are known for which no unifying explanation exists. For example, the penetrance of type I diabetes in the offspring of people with diabetes is higher when the father is the affected parent (Table 1.5) and when the paternal DR4-containing haplotypes are preferentially passed to the offspring.

Autoantibodies and Autoantigens

The identification of circulating ICAs in diabetic and subsequently in nondiabetic first-degree relatives has made it possible to detect the preclinical disease. ICAs are usually of the IgG class and are detected in vitro by their binding to islet cells in unfixed, frozen pancreas section using indirect immunofluorescence. Most (65–85%) newly diagnosed patients with type I diabetes have circulating ICAs as do 2–3% of unaffected first-degree relatives. This latter group of ICA-positive individuals are at high risk for developing type I diabetes. The similarity in the frequency of autoimmune markers in families with more than one affected individual has been compelling; yet type I diabetes can occur in relatives without documented autoimmunity. Conversely, autoimmune markers may persist for ≥ 5 yr in some individuals without evidence of metabolic deterioration.

Early studies distinguished three types of ICAs: cytoplasmic, surface, and complement fixing. Heterogenicity exists in both the antigens and antibodies of islet cell autoimmunity. More recent studies have focused on the actual molecular identities. Excellent examples are insulin and the 64K antigen, now known to be a glutamic acid decarboxylase (GAD). Ganglioside components of the islet cell membrane and a protein with partial sequence homology to cow's milk protein are other potential candidate antigens. However, it is unclear whether the autoantibodies directed at GAD or any islet cell antigen are the cause or result of β-cell injury.

Most patients with type I diabetes have nonpancreatic, organ-specific autoantibodies (e.g., thyroid, gastric parietal cells, and less often, adrenal). Although Hashimoto's thyroiditis is the most common autoimmune disorder associated with type I diabetes, the range of organ involvement can vary from none to severe polyglandular failure. Conversely, only 6% of patients with nonpancreatic autoimmune endocrinopathies are ICA-positive; however, few of these individuals will actually progress to overt type I diabetes. Autoantibodies directed against insulin are found in 20–60% of patients with type I diabetes before the initiation of exogenous insulin therapy. They are particularly prevalent among those patients with a younger age of disease onset. The combination of high-titer ICA, insulin autoantibodies, and decreased first-phase insulin secretion is predictive of the onset of type I diabetes within 5 yr.

Screening and Intervention Trials

Humoral autoantibodies allow for the identification of individuals who are at high risk for developing type I diabetes, and they may also play a role in experimental, therapeutic trials directed at the preservation of islet cell function. Screening for immunologic markers of type I diabetes in any population outside the context of defined research studies is discouraged. Screening of high-risk individuals (e.g., 1st-degree relatives of someone with type I diabetes) should be encouraged providing that individuals who screen positive are referred to centers participating in cooperative intervention studies or other scientific investigations using appropriate techniques. All subjects who are screened but do not enter a study should be counseled about their risk of developing diabetes, and follow-up should be offered.

Cell-Mediated Immunologic Dysfunction

The existence of insulitis (lymphocytic infiltration of the pancreas by mononuclear cells) has been known for decades and was the earliest evidence for the autoimmune nature of type I diabetes. There is evidence of a role for both T and B lymphocytes as well as lymphokines in the pathophysiology of the β-cell destruction in both human and animal models. However, type I diabetes in most animal models is considered a cell-mediated disease because adoptive transfer occurs with T lymphocytes but

Table 1.5. Approximate Familial Risk of Type I Diabetes

RELATIONSHIP TO PROBAND	RISK (%)
Sibling	6
Identical twin	25–50
HLA	
Identical	15
Haploidentical	6
Nonidentical	1
Father	6
Mother	1
Offspring	5
General population	0.4

Adapted from Muir A, Schatz DA, Maclaren NK: The pathogenesis, prediction, and prevention of insulin-dependent diabetes mellitus. *Endocrin Metab Clin North Am* 21:201, 1992

not with autoantibody transfer. Therapies directed against T lymphocytes are more successful than antibody-depleting treatments such as plasmapheresis.

Environmental Triggers

The concordance rate of diabetes of identical twins suggests that environmental factors may be important in the pathogenesis of type I diabetes. Viral infections, e.g., Coxsackie B4 and congenital rubella, have been inconsistently implicated as triggers for the immunological process. Exposure to substances toxic to the β-cells accounts for only a very small number of cases. Prolonged breastfeeding is reported to lower the incidence rates for type I diabetes. Little direct evidence exists to link any specific factor(s) to triggering autoimmune destruction of the β-cells in type I diabetes in humans.

CONCLUSION

Individuals who are genetically or otherwise predisposed to develop type I diabetes eventually demonstrate near total failure of insulin secretion as the result of an immunologically mediated progressive destruction of β-cell mass. The emergence of insulinopenia is associated with several intracellular abnormalities in both liver and muscle tissue, leading to excessive hepatic glucose production, decreased muscle glucose uptake, frank glucose intolerance, and if untreated, ketoacidosis. Because insulin deficiency is primary, patients are dependent on exogenous insulin for life.

BIBLIOGRAPHY

Barrett E, DeFronzo RA: Diabetic ketoacidosis. *Hosp Pract* 19:89–104 1984

Eisenbarth GS: Type I diabetes mellitus: a chronic autoimmune disorder. *N Engl J Med* 314:1360–68, 1986

Eisenbarth GS, Connelly J, Soeldner JS: The "natural" history of type I diabetes. *Diabetes Metab Rev* 3:873–92, 1987

Eisenbarth GS, DiMario U (Eds.): Immunotherapy of insulin-dependent diabetes mellitus. *Diabetes Spectrum* 5:267–305, 1992

Gepts W, In't Veld PA: Islet morphologic changes. *Diabetes Metab Rev* 3:859–72, 1987

Lernmark A: Molecular biology of type I (insulin-dependent) diabetes mellitus. *Diabetologia* 28:195–203, 1985

Muir A, Schatz DA, Maclaren NK: The pathogenesis, prediction and prevention of insulin-dependent diabetes mellitus. *Endocrin Metab Clin North Am* 21:199–219, 1992

Nerup J, Mandrup-Poulsen T, Molvig J: The HLA-IDDM association: implications for etiology and pathogenesis of IDDM. *Diabetes Metab Rev* 3:779–802, 1987

Palmer JP, McCulloch DK: Prediction and prevention of IDDM—1991. *Diabetes* 40:943–47, 1991

Riley WJ, Winter WE, Maclaren NK: Identification of insulin-dependent diabetes mellitus before onset of clinical symptoms. *J Pediatr* 112:314–16, 1988

Routine Management: Objectives

Highlights

Philosophy and Goals

Diabetes Self-Management Education

Highlights
Routine Management: Objectives

PHILOSOPHY AND GOALS

Three factors that strongly influence treatment are
- the health-care team's treatment philosophy, including beliefs regarding glycemic control and complications
- the patient's self-care attitudes and abilities, and
- physician-patient congruence of goals.

The primary goals of treatment are
- to promote and maintain day-to-day clinical and psychological well-being;
- to avoid severe hypoglycemia, symptomatic hyperglycemia, and ketoacidosis, and
- to promote normal growth and development in children.

Results from the Diabetes Control and Complications Trial demonstrated a link between glycemic control and development of diabetic complications.

Strong experimental support for an association between metabolic abnormalities and vascular complications is found in animal studies.

The physician and patient must set treatment goals together with the health-care team and family. Glycemic goals should be set as close to normal as possible given the patient's abilities and presence of risk factors.

Initial and long-term clinical goals are presented on page 18. They focus on
- metabolic stabilization
- restoration and maintenance of desirable body weight, and
- elimination of hyperglycemic symptoms.

DIABETES SELF-MANAGEMENT EDUCATION

The goal of diabetes self-management education is to provide patients with the knowledge, skills, and motivation to incorporate diabetes self-management into their daily life. To meet this goal, diabetes education must provide
- teaching of information needed for diabetes self-management
- training in skills needed for treatment procedures
- guidance on devising methods to fit the treatment regimen into the individual's lifestyle, and
- counseling on reconciling diabetes care and the individual's view of quality of life.

Diabetes self-management education is a planned process that includes
- an assessment to identify the patient's individual education needs
- planning specific education strategies
- implementation and documentation of education, and
- evaluation of effectiveness.

To be effective, patient education must be individualized, should be provided in a team approach to diabetes care, and needs to continue across the lifespan of the individual with diabetes.

Newly diagnosed patients with type I diabetes need to learn the basic skills that will enable them to implement their treatment regimen at home. Initial education should focus on teaching survival skills with more in-depth information and additional topics added after the patient has had time to adjust to diabetes self-management. Written patient guidelines for detecting and treating hypoglycemia and for managing mild illnesses reinforce self-management skills that are not routinely needed.

Patient education is essential for management of type I diabetes. Therefore, physicians who treat type I patients need to provide diabetes self-management training. Physicians can incorporate diabetes patient education in their clinical practice by
- hiring diabetes educators

- developing a team relationship with diabetes educators working in the community, and
- referring patients to diabetes education programs recognized by the American Diabetes Association as meeting the National Standards for Diabetes Patient Education Programs.

Philosophy and Goals

INTRODUCTION

Insulin-dependent (type I) diabetes mellitus is a chronic disease in which the goals and attitudes of the health-care team together with those of the patient are paramount in determining management and outcome. The health-care team comprises a consortium that includes the endocrinologist, nurse, dietitian, social worker, mental health professional, and medical specialists. Three factors that strongly influence treatment are

- the health-care team's treatment philosophy, including beliefs regarding glycemic control and complications
- the patient's self-care attitudes and abilities, and
- physician-patient congruence of goals.

The primary goals of treatment are *1)* to promote and maintain day-to-day clinical and psychological well-being; *2)* to avoid severe hypoglycemia, symptomatic hyperglycemia, and ketoacidosis; and *3)* to promote normal growth and development in children. The secondary goal of treatment is to provide the patient with the necessary tools to achieve the best possible glycemic control to prevent, delay, or arrest the micro- and macrovascular complications while minimizing hypoglycemia and excess weight gain. The primary goals are clearly achievable at reasonable degrees of cost, inconvenience, and risk; the secondary goal, although more difficult, should be attainable by most patients.

GLYCEMIC CONTROL AND COMPLICATIONS: A SUMMARY OF EVIDENCE

Evidence relating hyperglycemia and/or other metabolic consequences of insulin deficiency to the development of vascular complications comes from older epidemiologic studies of European and North American patients with type I diabetes and from more recent controlled clinical trials from Scandinavia and North America. The Diabetes Control and Complications Trial (DCCT), sponsored by the National Institutes of Health was, a long-term, prospective, randomized, controlled, multicenter trial that studied the course of approximately 1400 patients with type I diabetes. The patients were treated with intensive or conventional insulin regimens. The DCCT was designed to answer two questions: *1)* whether intensive glycemic control could prevent microvascular disease from developing, and *2)* whether it could arrest or reverse early microvascular complications already present (with retinopathy as the primary endpoint). The study found that there is a link between glycemic control and development of diabetic complications. Intensively treated patients who achieve similar metabolic control can expect a 50–75% reduction in the risk of developing progression of retinopathy, nephropathy, and neuropathy after 8–9 yr. These changes begin to appear at 3–4 yr. Similar results have been reported in the smaller Stockholm Diabetes Intervention Study.

Prospective Clinical Trials

The DCCT examined whether intensive treatment with the goal of maintaining glucose concentrations close to the normal range could decrease the frequency and severity of diabetic complications. Investigators studied 1441 patients with type I diabetes—726 with no retinopathy and 715 with mild retinopathy at baseline. Patients were randomly assigned to intensive therapy administered with insulin pumps or multiple injections of insulin guided by blood glucose monitoring or to conventional therapy with one or two insulin injections per day. The patients were followed a mean of 6.5 yr. Results showed that in the primary intervention cohort, intensive therapy reduced the mean risk of developing retinopathy by 76%. In the secondary intervention group, intensive therapy slowed the progression of retinopathy by 54% and reduced the development of proliferative retinopathy by 47%. In both groups combined, intensive therapy reduced the occurrence of microalbuminuria (>40 mg/24 h) by 39% and albuminuria (>300 mg/24 h) by 54%. Clinical neuropathy was reduced by 60%. The most important adverse effect was a threefold increase in severe hypoglycemia. Comparable results were seen in the Stockholm Diabetes Intervention Study after 5 and 8 yr.

Animal Studies

Strong experimental support for an association between metabolic abnormalities and vascular complications is found in animal studies. Animals that are rendered insulin deficient and hyperglycemic develop pathologic changes resembling early human retinopathy, nephropathy, and neuropathy. These changes can be prevented or ameliorated and, in some instances, even reversed by early intensive insulin treatment, by curing diabetes via pancreas transplantation, or by transplanting the affected organ into a nondiabetic animal.

Other Causes of Diabetes

Microvascular disease also develops in some patients with diabetes resulting from removal or destruction of the islets due to pancreatectomy, chronic pancreatitis, or toxicity (e.g., from the rodenticide Vacor). These observations further support the theory that loss of insulin secretion or some consequent metabolic derangement is responsible for microvascular abnormalities in patients with idiopathic type I diabetes. Genetic predisposition may influence the development of microvascular, neuropathic, and other complications; however, hyperglycemia is a prerequisite to development of these complications.

Kidney Transplantation Observations

Normal kidneys transplanted into recipients with type I diabetes begin to show pathologic changes resembling diabetic nephropathy after several years. Normal kidneys transplanted into patients with successful, whole-pancreas transplanta-tion have less glomerulopathy than kidneys transplanted into patients treated with conventional therapy. These observations point to a causative role for the diabetic metabolic milieu.

Epidemiologic Studies

Several epidemiologic studies in patients with type I diabetes suggest that the higher the glucose level, the greater the incidence of microvascular disease.

GOALS OF TREATMENT

The physician and patient, with the health-care team and family, must set treatment goals together. If overlooked, this deceptively simple point often leads to failure. The physician convinced of the importance of targeted glycemic control in every case will be frustrated by a patient who does not understand the need for, or is unable to accept the goal or methods used to, achieve glycemic control. Conversely, the patient who wants blood glucose levels to be normal all the time and is truly willing to work for it will be frustrated by a physician who lacks the time, facilities, conviction, or training to help achieve this goal or who is unable to guide the patient to achieve a safe and realistic set of goals.

In addition to a clear agreement on goals, a good health-care team–patient treatment match requires open communication and appropriate patient education. At the tightest end of the treatment spectrum, the patient must have a sophisticated and practical understanding of physiology and pharmacology when striving to maintain normal glucose levels when, for example, exercising strenuously. In contrast, at the looser end, knowledge may be more rudimentary, but patients must at least know that to avoid diabetic ketoacidosis (DKA), they may have to take extra insulin on sick days when appetite is poor and common sense seems to dictate the reverse. Treatment must always be individualized with regard to specific goals. Goals should be realistic and achievable. Success in achieving small incremental steps is more likely to lead to a larger goal. Sometimes more can be gained by striving for less.

The physician and other team members should avoid seeming autocratic, moralistic, or judgmental. They should try to be understanding when goals are not met easily or quickly and should empathize with the patient's difficulty in paying daily attention to the neverending demands of diabetes. It may help to work with the patient to identify obstacles to the treatment plan so the patient can address them. It is important to encourage the best goals achievable without demanding the impossible, unsafe, or impractical.

CLINICAL GOALS

Initial Goals

For the new-onset, acutely decompensated patient or the previously diagnosed patient in poor control, goals should include
- elimination of ketosis
- a return to desirable body weight range by reversing water and extracellular electrolyte losses and replenishing lean body mass (protein and intracellular electrolytes)
- elimination of obvious consequences of hyperglycemia, e.g., gross polyuria and polydipsia, vaginitis or balanitis, recurrent infections, and visual blurring due to reversible refractive changes, and
- avoid cerebral edema in cases of DKA.

Additional Goals

Once the initial clinical goals have been achieved, additional goals should include
- preventing symptoms of hyperglycemia, such as excessive thirst and urinary frequency, from disturbing sleep, school, work, social, or recreational activities
- preventing spontaneous and illness-induced ketosis
- maintaining weight within a desirable range

- stimulating catch-up growth and sexual maturation in children with poor glycemic control
- maintaining normal growth rate in children and adolescents
- maintaining maximum exercise tolerance and stamina
- maintaining a sense of psychosocial well-being and normal initiative in self-management
- minimizing self-treatable hypoglycemia and avoiding severe hypoglycemic seizures, accidents (e.g., while driving), and coma
- avoiding hospitalization
- for women, achieving normal fertility and pregnancy outcome
- sustaining normal family and marital relationships and sex life, and
- preventing diabetes-dictated or diabetes-oriented lifestyle (i.e., diabetes controlling the patient rather than vice versa).

LEVELS OF CONTROL

In addition to the educational and clinical goals discussed above, patients and the health-care team should individualize glycemic control goals. The results of treatment may be characterized in terms of three broad levels of control—minimal, average, and intensive—each having a typical biochemical and clinical profile (Table 2.1). Minimal control is unacceptable under all normal circumstances. In cases of average control, improvement should be attempted if the patient's clinical and personal situations permit. It is desirable to aim for intensive control, if it can be achieved without significant serious side effects. All patients should be given the opportunity to pursue more intensive diabetes treatment strategies, based on an assessment of potential risks and benefits.

Assessors of Control

Diabetes control is assessed by the patient at home via self-monitoring of blood glucose (SMBG) and urine ketones. At the office, longer term glycemic control is assessed by results of glycohemoglobin tests. Glycated hemoglobin values are expressed in two ways corresponding to the most commonly available types of assays: hemoglobin A_{1c} (HbA_{1c}) and either HbA_1 or total glycated hemoglobin (GHb) (see MONITORING, page 55). In absolute terms, HbA_1 or GHb values are generally 1.0–2.0% greater than HbA_{1c} values; however, the slope of these two assays' relationship to mean blood glucose is not parallel. Generally, a 1% change in HbA_{1c} or HbA_1 levels corresponds to a change in mean blood glucose of 35 mg/dl (1.9 mM). In nondiabetic individuals, HbA_{1c} values are 4.0–6.0%, whereas GHb values are 5.0–8.0%. These correspond to mean blood glucose levels of ~90 mg/dl (~5 mM).

When data compiled from diabetes specialty clinics in North America and Europe are analyzed, patients with type I diabetes show median HbA_{1c} values of 8.0–9.0% and GHb values of 10.0–11.0%. These correspond to mean blood glucose levels of ~200 mg/dl (~11.1 mM). Adolescents with type I diabetes generally average 0.5–1.0% higher values and a blood glucose that is 20–40 mg/dl (1.1–2.2 mM) higher than adults. Ninety-five percent of type I patients have an HbA_{1c} of 5.0–13.0% and a GHb of 6.0–15.0%. Levels as high as 20–25% are seen in the newly diagnosed and patients with very poor glycemic control.

Patients with hemoglobin variants (HbS, C, F) cannot have their glucose control measured with HbA_{1c} or HbA_1 assays employing conventional high-performance liquid or cation exchange chromatography. In these patients, glucose control can be assessed with radioimmunoassay methods for measuring HbA_{1c} and affinity chromatography methods for GHb.

Glycemic Control Goals

The following levels of glycemic control are appropriate for patients with type I diabetes.
- In all pregnant women and women attempting to conceive, seek stringent biochemical goals of intensive treatment (5.5–6.5% HbA_{1c} and 5.5–7.0% GHb, blood glucose 60–120 mg/dl [3.3–6.7 mM]) by methods detailed below (see PREGNANCY, page 94).

Table 2.1. Levels of Treatment: Biochemical and Clinical Characteristics

Minimal (unacceptable under all normal circumstances)
- HbA_{1c} 11.0–13.0% and GHb 13.0–15.0%
- Many SMBG values >300 mg/dl (>16.7 mM)
- Intermittent ketonuria
- Mean blood glucose level >300 mg/dl (>16.7 mM)

Average (improvement should be attempted if the patient's clinical and personal situations permit)
- HbA_{1c} 8.0–9.0% and GHb 10.0–11.0%
- Premeal SMBG 160–200 mg/dl (8.9–11.1 mM)
- Rare ketonuria
- Mean blood glucose level 160–240 mg/dl (8.9–11.1 mM)

Intensive (desired, if possible to achieve without significant serious side effects)
- HbA_{1c} 6.0–7.0% and GHb 7.0–9.0%
- Premeal SMBG 80–120 mg/dl (4.4–6.7 mM)*
- Bedtime SMBG 100–140 mg/dl (5.6–7.8 mM)
- Essentially no ketonuria
- Mean blood glucose level 120–160 mg/dl (6.7–8.9 mM)

SMBG, self-monitoring of blood glucose.
*This goal is similar to the 70–120 mg/dl (3.9–6.7 mM) goal used in the Diabetes Control and Complications Trial. Over the course of this study, >75% of morning (fasting) glucose levels were >120 mg/dl (>6.7 mM). In practice, the majority of prebreakfast glucose levels will be between 80 and 160 mg/dl (4.4–8.9 mM) in patients with HbA_{1c} values <7.0% yet acceptable rates of severe hypoglycemia.

- In nonpregnant patients who are well-informed about the risks and potential benefits of intensive therapy and are highly motivated and suitably educable, seek an intensive level of control (6.0–7.0% HbA_{1c} and 7.0–9.0% GHb). This is accomplished with average blood glucose levels of 110–150 mg/dl (6.1–8.3 mM). These goals are sought if achievable without significant serious side effects. Day-to-day fluctuations in blood glucose level are unavoidable. If the patient does not sense or respond to hypoglycemia or has frequent severe hypoglycemia, goals should be set higher to reduce the risk of severe hypoglycemia.
- In all patients, seek at least the average level of treatment (8.0–9.0%

HbA$_{1c}$ and 10.0–11.0% GHb). Ideally, improvement should be attempted if the patient's clinical and personal situations permit even though this goal may not be achieved in all patients.

Results of Minimal Control

A minimal level of glycemic control may be the best that can be achieved in some patients. However, it should never be accepted as a goal unless efforts by the health-care team to improve control alienate the patient, make routine follow-up care impossible, and make emergency care the rule. (Note that because blood glucose levels tend to rise with age in nondiabetic subjects, the elderly patient with 8–9% HbA$_{1c}$ may be considered to be closer to an acceptable level of control than a younger patient.) Table 2.1 shows the acceptable biochemical findings for patients with type I diabetes.

With a minimal level of control, patients will have symptoms of polyuria and polydipsia (that may not be noticed or admitted to) and a growth pattern that is probably slower than would otherwise be genetically determined. On the other hand, at this level of control, DKA can usually be avoided, and patients can generally function in some fashion at home, work, or school.

Results of Average Control

With an average level of treatment, patients will experience little or no polyuria or polydipsia, maintain body weight, exhibit normal-range growth rates, and usually appear to function normally in daily living. They will probably average one self-treated hypoglycemic reaction per week, and 10% will suffer one severe reaction every year. Achieving at least this result ensures the patient of a state of acceptable clinical well-being and offers the satisfaction of knowing that this individual is doing better than half of all patients with type I diabetes.

Results of Intensive Control

At an intensive level of control, patients are entirely asymptomatic and may perceive very good or excellent sense of well-being, energy, and exercise capaci-

ty and less disease-related anxiety compared with maintenance at poor control. They may also express a greater sense of control over the management of the disease. However, they may experience increased mild, self-treated and also severe hypoglycemic episodes. Some patients may feel excessively burdened by the required frequent monitoring, insulin-administration methods, and constant dietary adherence. Negotiation (and renegotiation) of mutually acceptable goals will reduce the chances that patients will abandon reasonable self-care.

CONCLUSION

For patients with type I diabetes, the long-term benefits of intensive insulin treatment appear extremely promising. These benefits must be balanced in each patient against actual risks and costs. The health-care team together with the patient should set treatment goals on the basis of their own best judgment regarding individual patient capabilities and understanding.

BIBLIOGRAPHY

DCCT Research Group: The effect of intensive treatment of diabetes on the development and progression of long-term complications in insulin-dependent diabetes mellitus. *N Engl J Med* 329:977–86, 1993

Klein R, Klein BEK, Moss SE, David MD, DeMets DL: Glycosylated hemoglobin predicts the incidence and progression of diabetic retinopathy. *JAMA* 260:2864–71, 1988

Pirart J: Diabetes mellitus and its degenerative complications: a prospective study of 4,400 patients observed between 1947 and 1973. *Diabetes Care* 1:168–88, 252–63, 1978

Reichard P, Nilsson BY, Rosenqvist U: The effect of long-term intensified insulin treatment on the development of microvascular complications of diabetes mellitus. *N Engl J Med* 329:304–309, 1993

Santiago JV: Lessons from the Diabetes Control and Complications Trial. *Diabetes* 42:1549–54, 1993

Diabetes Self-Management Education

INTRODUCTION

Diabetes management is a team effort. Physicians, nurses, dietitians, and other health-care professionals contribute their expertise and long-term implementation to the design of therapeutic regimens that will enable patients to achieve the best possible metabolic control. The patient is at the center of the team and, supported by his or her family, has responsibility for day-to-day implementation of the treatment plan. In the case of children, the caregivers take on this responsibility. Therapy will be most effective if the patient understands the regimen, is not ambivalent about the value, and has mastered the skills to do required tasks correctly. Therefore, the clinical management of diabetes relies on patient self-management.

The importance of patient education is underscored by the Diabetes Control and Complications Trial, which demonstrated that intensive treatment of diabetes, with great demands in patient self-management, can prevent or delay the long-term complications of diabetes. Intensive therapy brings an increased risk of hypoglycemia, making patient education critical in providing safety. This section provides an overview of diabetes patient education, including information on the principles, process, content, and guidelines for incorporating education into clinical practice. Currently, several terms, including diabetes self-management education and diabetes self-management training, are being used to describe patient education in diabetes. They will be used interchangeably in this manual. However, for reimbursement purposes, diabetes self-management training is the preferred terminology.

GENERAL PRINCIPLES

The goal of diabetes self-management education is to provide patients with the knowledge, skills, and motivation to incorporate diabetes self-management into their daily life. To meet this goal, diabetes education must include teaching patients the new information they need to know about diabetes management, training them in the various skills they need for treatment procedures, assisting them in devising methods to fit the regimen into their lifestyle, and helping them reconcile diabetes care with their quality of life so they are motivated to manage their disease.

Ideally, a health-care team should be involved in patient education. Many physicians may not have a diabetes education team available in their practice setting and need to refer patients, if possible, to a diabetes education program or to diabetes educators. Physicians can develop a team approach by collaborating with nurses and dietitians working in community outpatient settings or in private practice. The local affiliate of the American Diabetes Association and the national office of the American Association of Diabetes Educators can provide names of certified diabetes educators. Also, the American Diabetes Association has identified diabetes education programs that meet the National Standards for Diabetes Patient Education Programs and will provide a list of recognized programs on request. This list is printed quarterly in *Diabetes Forecast.*

Diabetes self-management education is a planned process that requires time, materials, space, and professional expertise (Table 2.2). The knowledge and skills patients need to implement their treatment regimen cannot be acquired during a quick interaction on the day of diagnosis or in a single instructional session in a physician's office. Moreover, patient education is an ongoing component of diabetes care, not a one-time referral.

For the newly diagnosed patient, a staged approach to education should be used, with the initial teaching focused on the critical information that will enable the individual, or caregiver, to implement the regimen at home (Table 2.3). Once the patient is comfortable with the fundamental components of the

Table 2.2. The Process of Diabetes Self-Management Education

Assessment:	identify patient's individual education needs
Planning:	set goals for education based on the assessment and select teaching/learning strategies
Implementation:	provide the planned education in an environment that supports learning
Documentation:	document educational activities to inform other members of the diabetes treatment team and to record the care provided
Evaluation:	measure the impact of education by testing knowledge and skills and by evaluating behavioral and metabolic outcomes

regimen, teaching can be expanded to provide more in-depth information and to introduce additional topics. Continuing education across the lifespan provides opportunities for learning new management techniques and for making adjustments in the regimen to accommodate lifestyle changes.

To be effective, diabetes self-management education must be individualized. Teaching methods, however, need not be limited to individual instruction. Group classes and self-study methods can supplement individual instruction and offer advantages in meeting different learning styles and in efficient use of teaching time. Information from all sources must be consistent, whether provided by different health professionals or from diverse instructional materials. Therefore, all members of the treatment team need to be aware of the content of the education program.

SELF-MANAGEMENT EDUCATION PROCESS

Diabetes self-management education is a systematic procedure that starts with an assessment of individual educational needs to guide planning of teaching/learning strategies, followed by implementation of the plan and documentation of the process, and concluding with evaluation of the outcomes. Although terms may be different, the process mim- ics the traditional steps clinicians use to diagnose and treat patients. Understanding the commonalties of patient education and medical care facilitates integration of education into the clinical management of diabetes.

Assessment

The first step in the educational process is an assessment to provide physical, psychosocial, and educability data to determine an individual education plan. Information obtained in this assessment can guide both treatment and education decisions. For example, if assessment shows that the individual has limited learning skills, treatment with a simple insulin regimen versus a complex algorithm of dose adjustments would be appropriate, with educational strategies providing pictorial instruction materials, demonstration with return demonstration, and a plan for evaluating accurate performance at home.

The education assessment also focuses on the three key areas of the learning process: cognitive/knowledge, psychomotor/skills, and affective/attitude. To develop teaching strategies, the educator needs to evaluate each patient to determine specific knowledge that needs to be acquired; skills that need to be mastered; and personal attitudes toward diabetes, health care, and life that will influence that patient's self-management of diabetes.

As a general framework, the educational assessment should include:

- Demographic information: age, gender, level of education, occupation, and family status.
- Medical history: height; weight; blood pressure; blood glucose values (glycated hemoglobin, fasting plasma glucose, and self-monitoring results); blood lipid values; medications (prescribed and over-the-counter); allergies; other medical problems; and general health status, including smoking, alcohol consumption, sexual activity, and use of social drugs.
- Diabetes history: type of diabetes; duration of diabetes; current treatment plan, including medication,

Table 2.3. Basic Education at Diagnosis: Survival Skills

Topics and the critical knowledge and skills patients need to manage their diabetes at home include:

General facts: explain the need for daily insulin injections and that treatment of diabetes involves insulin, diet, exercise, and self-monitoring of blood glucose levels

Medications: measure insulin dosage accurately, inject correctly, understand timing of injections and how to handle insulin and supplies

Nutrition: explain the relationship of food, insulin and blood glucose, and the amount, type of food and times to eat to maximize blood glucose control

Exercise: explain the relationships of exercise, food, and insulin and how to prevent hypoglycemia from exercise

Monitoring: perform accurate self-monitoring of blood glucose (SMBG) and urine ketones

Hyperglycemia & hypoglycemia: differentiate the signs and symptoms of high and low blood glucose levels and know what actions to take for each situation; know when to seek immediate medical assistance for intercurrent illness, hyperglycemia, or ketonuria.

Use of the health-care system: identify how to obtain insulin supplies, whom to call for professional advice, and how to get help in an emergency

diet, exercise, monitoring, and problems with adherence; acute and chronic complications; family history; and previous diabetes education.
■ Dietary habits: meal times and locations, snacking patterns, food preferences, resources for food preparation, and previous diet instructions. (Note that nutrition therapy includes a more detailed history; see the section on Nutrition.)
■ Physical activity: work/school activity, recreational activity.
■ Social history: information on household, extended family, social network, cultural factors, religious practices, health beliefs, and current health practices.
■ Economic profile: income, insurance, transportation resources, and neighborhood environment.
■ Lifestyle: activities of daily living including work, school, and leisure time. For children, information on after-school, weekend, and summer activities.

■ Psychosocial status: feelings about diabetes, personal relationships (with spouse, partner, parents, family, peers), developmental stages in life-cycle, history of sleep or eating disorders, stress, anxiety, or depression.
■ Education factors: literacy, computational skills, readiness to learn, preferred learning methods, visual acuity, hearing loss, and dexterity.
Additional information will be required to develop educational plans to meet idiosyncratic needs of individual patients. Also, as with nutrition, each member of the treatment team will use a more extensive assessment specific to their area of expertise.

Planning Educational Strategies

The assessment identifies the topics that need to be included in the education plan and teaching methods that would be most effective. From this analysis, educational goals are developed for each patient. The educational goals must correspond with therapeutic goals established by the treatment team and diabetes management goals set by the patient. If the treatment team is focused on normalization of blood glucose and the patient is focused on making a minimum number of lifestyle changes, teaching will not be effective until there is agreement. Once goals are established, measurable, behavioral objectives are developed with the patient to clearly identify steps that will be used to achieve these goals.

The education plan delineates what is to be taught when, how, where, and by whom. There are a number of teaching strategies that can be used with a patient (Table 2.4). For a newly diagnosed patient, the plan would specify topics that need to be covered immediately to provide the patient with the "survival skills" necessary to manage his or her diabetes at home (Table 2.3). Teaching methods could include

- one-on-one sessions with the dietitian to develop a meal plan
- one-on-one sessions with the diabetes nurse educator to learn insulin injection and monitoring techniques
- observation of patient injection and monitoring skills by staff nurses
- a videotape describing pathophysiology
- group classes on balancing the insulin—diet—exercise triad and on preventing and treating hypoglycemia, and
- a case study with questions to evaluate learning and problem-solving skills.

The plan would include methods for evaluating learning accomplished in the initial phase, steps to reinforce what has been taught, and resources for obtaining in-depth education within a reasonable time frame.

Implementation

Teaching can take place in a classroom, at bedside, in an office, in the cafeteria, or in a number of other settings. Whatever space is used, it is critical that the environment support learning and reinforce the importance of the educational process. There should be adequate lighting and furnishings and minimal distractions. Education sessions should be scheduled at specific times. Scheduling will help assure that teaching takes place; deter the potential for tests, visitors, or other situations receiving priority; and establish the concept that education is a specific part of diabetes care. The same measures used to reinforce routine clinical appointments should be used including written information giving the appointment time, location (with directions if needed), and the name(s) and telephone number(s) of the educator(s).

Documentation

Documentation of education is as important as documentation of treatment procedures. Documentation provides a means of communication among healthcare team members as well as substantiating the provision of educational care. Documentation can be included in progress notes in the patient's medical chart, maintained in education charts, or written in correspondence and reports. Whatever method of documentation is used, a permanent record of a patient's educational experience must be maintained.

Evaluation

The effectiveness of the educational plan is evaluated in several ways. First, testing will provide measures of knowledge gained, skills acquired, and changes in attitudes. This type of evaluation often is included in the implementation process to allow for reinforcement in areas where the patient exhibits weaknesses. Periodic assessment will provide measures of lapses in knowledge, skills, or attitudes that can be remedied with a refresher course. Another evaluation procedure measures changes in behavior. This evaluation takes place some time after education (3–6 mo) to measure whether the behavior is being maintained. The behavioral objectives developed during the planning phase may be used, or a dif-

Table 2.4. Teaching Strategies

Methods
- Individual instruction: education can be tailored to individual learning needs and focused on specific details of patient's self-management plan
- Group classes: efficient use of educator time, patients benefit from social support and peer learning
- Self-study: flexible, allows patient to pace learning, educator should monitor and evaluate progress

Techniques
- Short lecture: effective for presenting new information
- Discussion: allows patient to personalize information, ask questions, disclose feelings, and share experiences
- Skills training: provides "hands on" learning; educator demonstrates, patient practices then demonstrates and receives feedback from educator
- Problem solving: allows patients to integrate information on several topics, such as diet, insulin, and exercise, and to test their knowledge in hypothetical situations
- Role playing: can be used to reinforce learning (patient plays educator role), to practice social skills (explaining diabetes to friends), and to explore personal problems (family stress)
- Case studies: provide an objective approach to learning that can be used for planning, problem solving, and to help patients identify errors they are making in their diabetes self-management
- Self-assessment: blood glucose records, food diaries, and exercise logs can be used to help patients recognize problems in their diabetes self-management and often to identify solutions.

Materials
- Printed materials: can be used to reinforce teaching, for self-study, and as an information resource for future needs (e.g., sick-day guidelines)
- Audio and visual aides: slides, films, overheads, audio and video tapes, food models and labels, sample diabetes products, and dolls and puppets are effective in enhancing learning
- Interactive learning programs: available in printed, audio, visual, and computer formats; allow individuals to learn at their own pace, with frequent evaluation to provide feedback on learning
- Games: crossword puzzles, board games, and group games introduce fun into the educational process while enhancing participant learning

ferent set of objectives can be set at the completion of education as an outgrowth of the learning process. A third approach evaluates the effectiveness of education by examining treatment goals such as lower glycated hemoglobin, minimal hypoglycemia, or absence of diabetic ketoacidosis. All forms of evaluation yield an assessment of additional educational needs of the patient.

CONTENT OF DIABETES SELF-MANAGEMENT EDUCATION

Topics to be included in diabetes patient education are numerous and vary according to type of diabetes, patient age, and other individual characteristics. The National Standards for Diabetes Patient Education Programs, published in 1983, specified that programs should be able to provide information in 15 content areas. In 1994, the Standards are being revised and the content areas modified to reflect current principles of diabetes self-management and of patient education. The suggested topics are listed below with basic teaching points for type I diabetes:

- **General facts.** Type I diabetes is a chronic metabolic disorder in which the body no longer produces insulin required to use food for energy. Lack of insulin can be life-threatening. Daily insulin injections are essential and need to be balanced with meals and exercise to manage diabetes.
- **Stress and psychosocial adjustment.** Fear, anger, and denial are common responses to the diagnosis

of diabetes. The day-by-day demands of diabetes management can be frustrating. Stress may cause problems with blood glucose control. Coping skills, stress reduction techniques, and professional counseling can help the patient handle the psychosocial impact of diabetes.

■ **Family involvement/social support.** Type I diabetes impacts the whole family. Family members, friends, co-workers, and teachers need to know about diabetes, how to support regimen adherence, and how to respond in case of emergencies.

■ **Nutrition.** Food is an important part of diabetes treatment and health. The amount, type and timing of meals and snacks must be balanced with insulin and exercise to maintain good blood glucose control. Meal plans should be individualized to reflect food preferences and daily schedules, provide optimum nutrition, and make diabetes self-management as effective as possible.

■ **Exercise/activity.** Exercise is recommended for health and diabetes management. Exercise and activity can affect blood glucose levels, usually by lowering them. Planning can prevent hypoglycemia that may occur during or after exercise.

■ **Medications.** Insulin must be taken daily as prescribed. It is important to know the type and amount of insulin to be taken, times to administer insulin, and to understand the action and duration of the prescribed insulin. Correct techniques for drawing up and injecting insulin are critical to assure that the dose is accurate. Glucagon is used to treat severe hypoglycemia. Family members and close friends need to know how to administer glucagon.

■ **Monitoring.** Proper technique is crucial to achieve reliable results. Blood glucose monitoring results can be used to assess the effectiveness of the treatment regimen, identify low blood glucose levels requiring treatment to prevent hypoglycemia, indicate high blood glucose levels

possibly associated with illness, show the effect of different meals and activities on blood glucose, and guide decisions on when to call health-care providers. Urine testing for ketones is required during times of physical or emotional stress.

■ **Relationships among nutrition, exercise, medication, and blood glucose levels.** Type I diabetes is treated by insulin, diet, and exercise. Understanding the interactions among the three and their impact on blood glucose levels is important in making self-management decisions. Self-monitoring values provide information that can be used to make adjustments in one or more of the three therapeutic agents.

■ **Prevention, detection, and treatment of acute complications (hypoglycemia, hyperglycemia, and illness).** Hypoglycemia comes on quickly. Therefore, it is important to recognize the signs and symptoms of hypoglycemia and to know how to prevent and treat it (Table 2.5). Hyperglycemia that cannot be explained by diet or another aspect of the regimen (e.g., decrease in exercise or inadequate insulin delivery or amount) may indicate illness. Patients with type I diabetes can develop diabetic ketoacidosis when ill. Therefore, guidelines for sick days need to be followed carefully (Table 2.6).

■ **Prevention, detection, treatment, and rehabilitation of chronic complications.** Chronic complications are a serious concern in diabetes. Steps that can reduce the risk of complications include maintaining blood glucose levels as near to normal as feasible, not smoking, having annual eye exams, controlling blood pressure and blood lipid levels, and taking preventive care of feet.

■ **Foot, skin, and dental care.** High blood glucose levels can lead to bacterial growth that can cause infections in many areas, including gums, skin, and feet. People with diabetes are also at risk for developing foot sores that they may not be aware of because of loss of sensation in their feet. Routine care to keep teeth, gums, and skin clean and to check feet for cuts and red or discolored areas is important.

■ **Behavior change strategies.** Most aspects of diabetes management require changes in behavior. Behavior change is not simply will-power. Techniques such as goal setting, contracting, and problem solving are helpful in changing habits to reduce health risks and improve diabetes control.

■ **Benefits, risks, and treatment options for improving blood glucose.** Achieving optimal blood glucose control may deter the complications of diabetes. However, tight control brings an increased risk of hypoglycemia. Individuals with diabetes need to be responsible for their diabetes management, which includes working with their health-care team to select the treatment plan that meets their personal goals for health.

■ **Preconception care and pregnancy.** Optimal blood glucose control will reduce risks to the infant in pregnancies complicated by diabetes. Women with type I diabetes need to achieve excellent blood glucose control before becoming pregnant (optimally for 3 mo before conception). Tight blood glucose control needs to be maintained throughout pregnancy.

■ **Use of health-care system/community resources.** People with diabetes need to be good consumers of the health-care system and of community resources. Ongoing versus episodic care is important. Telephone numbers of health-care team members and emergency services should be readily available for use by family and friends as well as the individual with diabetes. Identifying resources in the community for supplies, services, information, and support groups makes day-to-day diabetes management easier.

Table 2.5. Sample Patient Guidelines for Treating Mild Hypoglycemia: 15/15 Rule

If blood glucose falls below 70 mg/dl:
■ Eat 15 g carbohydrate
■ Wait 15 minutes—retest, and if blood glucose remains <70 mg/dl, treat with another 15 g carbohydrate
■ Repeat testing and treating until blood glucose returns to normal range
■ If >1 h to next meal, add additional 15 g carbohydrate to maintain blood glucose in normal range

Sources of carbohydrate—15-g portions

Glucose products:
Glucose tablet	3 tablets
Glutose	1-1/2 25-g tubes
Insta glucose	1/2 31-g tube
Monoject gel	1-1/2 25-g packets

Food/beverages:
LifeSavers	5
Jelly beans	6
Raisins	2 Tbsp.
Sugar or honey	1 Tbsp.
Juice (apple/orange)	1/2 cup
Soft drink (regular)	1/2 cup
Skim milk	1 cup
Ginger ale	3/4 cup

Note: Severe hypoglycemia needs to be treated by someone knowledgable about diabetes. Guidelines should be available in schools and worksites. If the patient cannot swallow well, glucagon must be used instead of oral treatment.

Additional Topics of Importance for Type I Diabetes

■ **Patient identification.** Wearing an identification bracelet or necklace at all times is strongly encouraged so that diabetes can be identified if severe hypoglycemia or an accident occurs.

■ **Driving a motor vehicle.** Special care should be taken to prevent hypoglycemia while driving a car, truck, motor boat, or any other powered vehicle. Blood glucose levels should be checked if the last meal was >3 h earlier or if the trip will be long and low blood glucose

Table 2.6. Sample Patient Guidelines for Sick-Day Management

Illness can make diabetes more difficult to manage. Even when you do not feel well, you must take your insulin, test blood glucose and urine ketones, drink fluids, and eat some food. You will need ketone strips and food such as regular gelatin and soft drinks. Therefore, planning ahead for sick days is important. The following guidelines will help you during mild illnesses.

Monitoring
Blood glucose and urine ketones need to be tested frequently during illness, often every 2–4 h. Test for ketones if you have unexplainable blood glucose values >250 mg/dl or if you feel ill, even if blood glucose values are normal. Write down the values and call a member of your health-care team when premeal blood glucose values stay >250 mg/dl and/or when you measure moderate or large ketones in the urine.

Insulin
Never stop taking insulin—even if vomiting and unable to eat. Your body often needs more insulin during illness. Therefore, your health-care professional may ask you to take supplemental insulin according to results of blood glucose monitoring.

Food and fluid intake
Use small meals and eat more frequently when you are ill. Soft foods or liquids are often tolerated best. Eating about 10–15 g of carbohydrate every 1–2 h is usually sufficient. Foods and beverages containing about 15 g carbohydrate include:

1/2 cup regular gelatin	3/4 cup regular gingerale
1/2 cup vanilla ice cream	1/2 cup regular soft drink
1/2 cup custard	1/2 cup orange or apple juice
1 regular double popsicle	1 cup Gatorade
1/2 cup applesauce	1 cup creamed soup

Fluid intake is essential during illness. If vomiting, diarrhea, or fever is presented take small quantities of liquids every 15–30 min. Clear broth, tea, and other fluids can supplement liquids containing carbohydrate.

Seek medical attention when you have:
■ fever >100° F
■ persistant diarrhea
■ vomiting and are unable to take fluids for ≥4 h
■ blood glucose levels that are difficult to control and/or ketones are found in urine (see information above on monitoring)
■ severe abdominal pain
■ other unexplained symptoms
■ illness that persists over 24 h

Physician's #_____   Pharmacy #_____

values treated appropriately (Table 2.5). Supplies for self-monitoring of blood glucose and treating hypoglycemia should be carried in the vehicle at all times. If symptoms of hypoglycemia occur, driving should stop immediately and not be resumed until blood glucose levels are in the normal range.

■ **Travel guidelines.** Insulin and diabetes supplies sufficient for the entire trip need to be carried with the traveler and not put into checked baggage. Food to treat hypoglycemia and for a meal that may be delayed by late arrival should be carried as well. Prescriptions for insulin and syringes should be taken along as well, in case the need to purchase supplies does occur.

■ **Career guidance.** Jobs that have erratic schedules, long periods between meals, lack the flexibility to stop work and test blood glucose levels, and other conditions make diabetes management more challenging. The Americans with Disabilities Act requires employers to make reasonable accommodations for employees with disabilities, including diabetes. The person with diabetes along with his or her supervisor and health-care team can identify ways to modify a job to accommodate the demands of work plus diabetes management.

INCORPORATING PATIENT EDUCATION IN CLINICAL PRACTICE

Patient education is essential for management of type I diabetes. However, all medical practice settings are not equipped to provide diabetes self-management training. Moreover, the complexity of type I diabetes, particularly when treated with intensive therapy, requires health-care providers to have special expertise in diabetes. Physicians who specialize in treatment of diabetes and who see many patients with type I diabetes can develop a team relationship with diabetes educators in the community, if hiring educators on a full- or part-time basis is not feasible. Systems such as health maintenance organizations, preferred provider organizations, and affiliations with hospitals offer potential resources for diabetes educators that can work with a number of physicians to maximize the economy of this specialized type of care. Physicians practicing in an area where there are programs recognized by the American Diabetes Association may refer patients to them, knowing that the programs meet the National Standards. The local American Diabetes Association Chapter or Affiliate maintains a listing of recognized programs in their area.

To establish a team approach to diabetes self-management education, the health professionals should *1*) share a common philosophy toward diabetes management, and *2*) develop efficient methods for communicating about patient care and education to assure that a consistent message is given to the patient. Forms can be helpful in documenting the educational process in a concise format that allows team members to keep abreast of each others' activities and to reinforce all areas of education. Sample forms can be found in the *Meeting the Standards* manual (see BIBLIOGRAPHY) and through networking with diabetes educators. Communication by fax and computers offers the opportunity for expedient transfer of information among health professionals not working in the same location. Forms, if placed in the front of a chart or a similar place routinely used in providing patient care, can serve as a prompt to educate while providing routine medical care.

Diabetes education materials can be obtained from the American Diabetes Association, from companies manufacturing pharmaceuticals and diabetes equipment and supplies, and through a number of additional resources available through the National Diabetes Information Clearinghouse.

CONCLUSION

Patients with type I diabetes need self-management education to be able to implement their treatment regimen. Education should be individualized to reflect the diabetes treatment regimen and learning characteristics of each patient. Self-management training is a systematic patient care process that requires educators with expertise in diabetes and resources in time and materials. Physicians should use a team approach to manage individuals with type I diabetes with self-management education integrated into the clinical care of the patient.

BIBLIOGRAPHY

A Core Curriculum for Diabetes Education. 2nd ed. Peragallo-Dittko V,

Ed. Chicago, IL, Am. Assoc. Diabetes Educators, 1993

American Diabetes Association position statement: Standards of medical care for patients with diabetes mellitus. *Diabetes Care* 17:616–24, 1994

Haire-Joshu D, Houston C: Promoting behavior change: teaching/learning strategies. In *Management of Diabetes Mellitus: Perspectives of Care Across the Life Span*. Haire-Joshu D, Ed. St. Louis, MO, Mosby, 1992, p. 565–92

Krall LP: Education: a treatment for diabetes. In *Joslin's Diabetes Mellitus*. 12th ed. Marble A, Krall LP,

Bradley RF, Christlieb AR, Soeldner JS, Eds. Philadelphia, PA, Lea & Febiger, 1985, p. 465–84

Meeting the Standards: A Manual for Completing the American Diabetes Association Application for Recognition. 3rd ed. Alexandria, VA, Am. Diabetes Assoc., 1991

Michigan Diabetes Research and Training Center: *Life With Diabetes: A Series of Teaching Outlines*. 3rd ed. Ann Arbor, MI, Univ. Michigan, 1991

Therapy for Diabetes Mellitus and Related Disorders. 2nd ed. Lebovitz HE, Ed. Alexandria, VA, Am. Diabetes Assoc., 1994

Routine Management: Tools

Highlights
Routine Management: Tools

INSULIN TREATMENT

Patients with type I diabetes are dependent on insulin to survive.

Insulin preparations are classified by species (beef, pork and, human) and duration of action (short, intermediate, and long acting) (Table 3.1).

Highly purified animal or human insulin is associated with fewer insulin antibodies, less insulin allergy, and less lipoatrophy at the injection site. Most newly diagnosed patients are started on human insulin.

The insulin regimen should be tailored to the needs of the individual patient. Therapy adjustments should be based on actual glycemic values obtained from patient self-monitoring of blood glucose (SMBG) rather than on "textbook" predictions of insulin action.

Single-injection regimens are usually inadequate in treating type I diabetes. Twice-daily insulin injections should be started as soon as possible after diagnosis. The two doses may consist of
■ intermediate-acting insulin alone, or
■ a flexible split-mixed short- and intermediate-acting insulin.

Other more intensive insulin regimens consist of
■ three or more daily injections, or
■ insulin infusion pump therapy.

Insulin needs may fluctuate during the first weeks or months of treatment. If a honeymoon phase occurs, insulin dose must be appropriately reduced, occasionally to as little as 0.1–0.3 U kg^{-1} day^{-1}, but should usually not be discontinued or replaced with an oral hypoglycemic agent.

Regimens employing insulin algorithms place more demands on both patient and physician than a fixed course of treatment. All forms of

intensive therapy require high degrees of long-term commitment and flexibility on the part of the patient, the family, and the health-care team.

Completely normal blood glucose values are extremely difficult to obtain except under rigorous research conditions.

Instructions for intensifying insulin therapy are found in Table 3.5. Continuous subcutaneous insulin infusion (pages 41–43) is an alternative that offers advantages in lifestyle flexibility despite physical, psychological, financial, and practical day-by-day burdens.

Common problems associated with insulin therapy are detailed on page 47.

MONITORING

Patients can only manage their diabetes effectively and safely if they are able to perform SMBG.

Monitoring allows objective goals for therapy and a means to measure the efficacy of changes in therapy.

Urine testing is easy and inexpensive. However, urine glucose tests cannot provide information about blood glucose in the acceptable or hypoglycemic range. Urine testing is the only practical way to detect ketones (acetone). All patients must test urine for ketones during illness or persistent hyperglycemia.

SMBG is the only monitoring method that allows
■ detection and prevention of hypoglycemia, and
■ adjustment of insulin, diet, and exercise to achieve target blood glucose levels.

Two SMBG measurements every day—before breakfast and supper—

provide the minimal information sufficient to adjust insulin and diet. Additional tests are needed at bedtime to minimize the occurrence of nocturnal hypoglycemia, when exercising, on sick days, or when schedule has changed (Table 3.7).

Common errors in SMBG include an inadequate drop of blood on the strip, poor technique in removing the blood from the strip, inaccurate timing, or incorrect or biased readings of "visually read" strips.

A properly performed glycated hemoglobin assay provides the best available index of chronic glucose levels. It is highly reliable and virtually tamperproof.

NUTRITION

The overall goal of nutritional management for type I diabetes is to enable patients to attain blood glucose levels as near normal as possible by integrating exogenous insulin into their usual eating and activity patterns. Recommendations depart from previous ones in not specifying the ideal macronutrient composition of the diet for diabetes but advocating that the diet prescription be individualized based on nutrition assessment and treatment goals. In general, recommendations follow nutrition guidelines for the general population:

■ Calorie levels should be prescribed to achieve and maintain reasonable body weight.
■ Protein intakes of 10–20% of calories are adequate to support health; intakes of 0.8 g/kg (10%) are recommended for individuals showing evidence of diabetic nephropathy.
■ Fat consumption should be moderate, with saturated fat limited to <10% of calories.
■ Carbohydrate foods such as grains, vegetables, and fruits are rich sources of vitamins, minerals, and dietary fiber, and a liberal intake is encouraged. Sugars differ from starches in

nutrient content but not in glycemic effect. For type I diabetes, the total amount of carbohydrate in a meal, rather than the source, should guide estimation of insulin dosage.
■ Vitamin and mineral requirements of individuals with diabetes are the same as the general population. Supplementation is advised if conditions create a deficiency.

Type I diabetes is easier to manage when people follow a consistent schedule and meals and insulin regimens are synchronized. Intensive insulin therapy, using multiple daily doses of insulin, allows greater flexibility in eating patterns than conventional therapy. Blood glucose levels obtained by self-monitoring can be used to make adjustments in diet and insulin regimen to maximize blood glucose control.

The complexity of integrating nutrition and insulin therapies and the importance of diabetes self-management education require a coordinated team approach to care of individuals with type I diabetes.

Diabetes nutrition therapy is based on an assessment of the individual's metabolic and lifestyle parameters, implemented through a nutrition self-management plan, and evaluated through nutrition-related outcomes such as blood glucose and lipid levels. Patients and their families should be actively involved in setting nutrition goals, developing the self-management plan, and in evaluating treatment effectiveness through self-monitoring of blood glucose levels.

Registered dietitians have the expertise to design the nutrition intervention and to counsel patients on nutrition self-management. Nutritional counseling for newly diagnosed patients with type I diabetes should be provided in stages to allow the patient time to adjust to the treatment regimen. Nutritional care cannot be limited to diagnosis but must continue throughout the patient's life span. Follow-up may be appropriate every 3–6 mo for children and every 6–12 mo for adults.

EXERCISE

Exercise should be an integral part of the treatment plan for patients with type I diabetes.

Physiological responses to exercise in nondiabetic people and in patients with type I diabetes are described in Table 3.14. For the type I patient, plasma insulin levels during and after exercise are critical determinants of response.

Potential benefits of exercise are explained on page 67. Regular exercise improves cardiovascular risk factors and may
■ aid in weight control, and
■ heighten sense of well-being.

Potential risks of exercise include destabilization of metabolic control, e.g.,
■ hypoglycemia during or after exercise (most likely with sporadic exercise); and

■ hyperglycemia to the point of ketoacidosis (if diabetes is controlled at a minimal level or blood glucose is high before beginning activity). Other risks of exercise are described on pages 68–69.

A preexercise medical evaluation should be performed regardless of the patient's age.

Exercise should be prescribed with caution in patients with
■ minimally controlled blood glucose;
■ cardiovascular disease, neuropathy that results in loss of sensation, or proliferative retinopathy; or
■ hypoglycemia unawareness.

Guidelines for safe exercise are addressed in Table 3.16. They include
■ monitoring blood glucose and taking appropriate action,
■ altering food or insulin if needed,
■ carrying short-acting carbohydrate and identification,
■ monitoring intensity of exercise, and
■ avoiding trauma to joints, muscle, or ligaments as well as to the skin of the feet.

Insulin Treatment

INTRODUCTION

Insulin-dependent (type I) diabetes mellitus is characterized by a near-absolute deficiency in endogenous insulin secretion within days or months after initial diagnosis. Affected patients are dependent on exogenous insulin to survive for the duration of their lives. Insulin injections are the mainstay of treatment and must be individualized for each patient.

INSULIN PREPARATIONS

Insulin preparations are generally classified by species (beef, pork, and human) and duration of action (short, intermediate, and long acting). Many insulin preparations are available; as a practical matter, health professionals should familiarize themselves with several of them and learn to use them rationally (Tables 3.1 and 3.2).

Species and Purity

Highly purified insulins of animal origin are now standard and contain less than one part per million of impurities and are associated with a reduced incidence of insulin antibodies, less insulin allergy, and less lipoatrophy at the injection site than previous preparations. Human insulin, prepared by recombinant DNA techniques, is also highly purified and is largely replacing animal insulins in the United States.

Like all foreign proteins, animal insulins are antigenic. Beef insulin differs from the human molecule by two amino acids, making it more antigenic than pork, which differs by only one amino acid. Human insulin, available only in highly purified form, is the least antigenic insulin available.

The clinician should be aware that human insulin may act quicker, peak earlier, and last a shorter time than animal insulins. Lipoatrophy at the injection site, probably related to impurities, may be prevented with either human or pure pork preparations.

It is still unclear whether all patients using animal insulins should change to pure pork or human insulin. Generally, patients started on one type of insulin should be maintained on it as long as they are doing well. Most newly diagnosed patients are started on human insulin. In the future, human insulin will probably replace all other currently available types. Rarely, pork NPH or ultralente insulins may be required for optimal nocturnal insulin replacement in patients with type I diabetes.

Duration of Action

Although insulins are classified into short-, intermediate-, and long-acting preparations, actual insulin effects do not always coincide with such simple descriptions. For example, local subcutaneous tissue conditions not clearly understood may cause rates of absorption to vary by 20–40% from day-to-day in any one patient. In light of the many other variables influencing insulin pharmacokinetics, the clinician is cautioned against relying too heavily on textbook descriptions of insulin action. Health professionals should base therapy adjustments on actual glycemic values obtained from the patient's self-monitoring of blood glucose (SMBG).

Any change in the dose of intermediate-acting (NPH) insulin requires a 2- to 5-day observation period before further dose adjustment because of the relatively slow absorption of these insulins and because of day-to-day variability in food, activity, and stress. An even longer period of observation is needed for long-acting preparations such as ultralente insulins.

The use of SMBG to map out a profile of blood glucose values is invaluable in assisting the physician, patient, and health-care team with therapy. Blood glucose levels should be measured before and after meals and several times during the night, particularly when initiating or intensifying insulin therapy or when seeking the cause of hypoglycemia or hyperglycemia. Routine frequency of

Table 3.1. Insulins Sold in the United States

PRODUCT	MANUFACTURER	STRENGTH
Short acting (usual onset 0.5–2.0 h; usual duration 3–6 h)		
Human		
Humulin regular	Lilly	U-100
Novolin R (regular)	Novo Nordisk	U-100
Velosulin human (regular)	Novo Nordisk	U-100
Novolin R Penfill (regular)	Novo Nordisk	U-100
Pork		
Iletin II regular	Lilly	U-100, U-500
Purified pork R (regular)	Novo Nordisk	U-100
Regular	Novo Nordisk	U-100
Beef/Pork		
Iletin I (regular)	Lilly	U-100
Intermediate acting (usual onset 3–6 h; usual duration 12–20 h)		
Human		
Humulin L (lente)	Lilly	U-100
Humulin N (NPH)	Lilly	U-100
Novolin L (lente)	Novo Nordisk	U-100
Novolin N (NPH)	Novo Nordisk	U-100
Novolin N Penfill (NPH)	Novo Nordisk	U-100
Beef		
NPH	Novo Nordisk	U-100
Lente	Novo Nordisk	U-100
Pork		
Iletin II Lente	Lilly	U-100
Iletin II NPH	Lilly	U-100
Purified pork lente	Novo Nordisk	U-100
Purified pork N (NPH)	Novo Nordisk	U-100
Beef/pork		
Iletin I Lente	Lilly	U-100
Iletin I NPH	Lilly	U-100
Long acting (usual onset 6–12 h; usual duration 18–36 h)		
Human		
Humulin U (Ultralente)	Lilly	U-100
Beef		
Ultralente	Novo Nordisk	U-100
Premixed combinations		
Human		
Humulin 50/50 (50% NPH, 50% regular)	Lilly	U-100
Humulin 70/30 (70% NPH, 30% regular)	Lilly	U-100
Novolin 70/30 (70% NPH, 30% regular)	Novo Nordisk	U-100
Novolin 70/30 Penfill	Novo Nordisk	U-100
Novolin 70/30 Prefilled	Novo Nordisk	U-100

monitoring should be based on mutually defined goals described in PHILOSOPHY AND GOALS (pages 17–18).

Mixing Insulins

The action-prolonging substances in intermediate- or long-acting insulin (NPH, lente, and ultralente) can sometimes affect the onset, peak, and duration of effectiveness of short-acting insulin in a mixture. Generally, the longer the contact time between the two types of insulin and the larger the proportion of intermediate- or longer-acting insulin in the mixture, the less rapid absorption of the short-acting insulin. Therefore, blood glucose levels fall at a slower rate, but the effect lasts longer. NPH may have a less pronounced effect on comixed regular insulin than do the lente insulins.

Mixing regular insulin with NPH in the same syringe is an accepted and convenient way to produce differently timed pharmacologic actions with a single injection. Similarly, semilente can be

Table 3.2. Insulins by Relative Comparative Action

INSULIN	ONSET (h)	PEAK (h)	EFFECTIVE DURATION (h)	MAXIMUM DURATION (h)
Animal				
Regular	0.5–2.0	3–4	4–6	6–8
NPH	4–6	8–14	16–20	20–24
Lente	4–6	8–14	16–20	20–24
Ultralente	8–14	Minimal	24–36	24–36
Human				
Regular	0.5–1.0	2–3	3–6	4–6
NPH	2–4	4–10	10–16	14–18
Lente	3–4	4–12	12–18	16–20
Ultralente	6–10	None	18–20	20–30

mixed with lente to improve the short-acting effect. (Lente is a mixture of 70% ultralente and 30% semilente.) It is not advisable to mix lente with regular insulin because it may alter the time course of the individual insulins. Stable premixtures of intermediate- and short-acting insulin in fixed proportion (e.g., 70% NPH/30% regular) are also available commercially. Premixed insulins are not suitable when daily variation in the dose of short-acting insulin is required.

TREATING NEWLY DIAGNOSED PATIENTS

Diagnosis and Stabilization

At diagnosis, initial objectives of therapy are eliminating symptomatic hyperglycemia (and concomitant fluid and electrolyte imbalance) while avoiding hypoglycemia. Therefore, glycemic targets should be approached gradually. Treatment should begin with approximately 0.6–0.75 $U \cdot kg^{-1} \cdot day^{-1}$. However, during the first week of therapy, this amount can be expected to increase to an average of 1 $U \cdot kg^{-1} \cdot day^{-1}$, because most patients are relatively insulin resistant at this time. This is particularly true for adolescents.

Immediately after diagnosis or after ketoacidosis has been resolved, therapy should begin with twice-daily insulin injections. It is preferable to start with the twice-daily regimen from the outset instead of spending several days using regular insulin every 4–6 h. Although once-daily insulin may suffice for a short time in patients who retain some β-cell function, psychological acceptance of twice-daily injections is easier for both patient and family if introduced as soon as possible after diagnosis, even if glycemic control could be adequate on one injection per day. About two-thirds of the insulin dose is given in the morning before breakfast, and one-third is given before supper. The two doses may consist of intermediate-acting insulin alone (usually this is the case for infants and very young children) or two doses of a mixture of short- and intermediate-acting insulins. The prebreakfast dose consists of about 2/3 NPH and 1/3 regular. The presupper dose is usually divided into equal amounts of NPH and regular insulin.

Patients and families should be taught the technique of blood glucose monitoring at diagnosis. They should determine blood glucose levels repeatedly under professional supervision to ensure the reliability of the readings. Although premixed formulations (e.g., 70% NPH/30% regular; 50% NPH/50% regular) may work satisfactorily in some patients under very stable control, all patients should have supplies of regular- and longer-acting insulins for use when needed.

Honeymoon Phase

Within weeks after diagnosis there may be some recovery of β-cell function, and consequently, exogenous insulin requirements often decrease for a period of weeks to months. This honeymoon phase of type I diabetes may be marked by the appearance of recurrent hypoglycemic reactions. A honeymoon phase occurs less frequently in younger children; it is more common in the late teenage years and in adults. During this period, insulin dosage must be appropriately reduced, occasionally to as little as $0.1–0.3 \text{ U} \cdot \text{kg}^{-1} \cdot \text{day}^{-1}$. Not all patients exhibit a profound honeymoon phase, but some period of stability in blood glucose levels is common, with insulin requirements at $0.2–0.5 \text{ U} \cdot \text{kg}^{-1} \cdot \text{day}^{-1}$. Evidence suggests that the honeymoon phase could be prolonged if blood glucose levels are kept within the near-euglycemic range.

Chronic Phase: Developing a Long-Term Treatment Plan

As the honeymoon period comes to an end with the progressive decrease of β-cell function, insulin requirements increase gradually over a period of several months. Prepubertal children usually require between 0.6 and $0.9 \text{ U} \cdot \text{kg}^{-1} \cdot \text{day}^{-1}$, and pubertal children may require up to $1.5 \text{ U} \cdot \text{kg}^{-1} \cdot \text{day}^{-1}$ due to relative insulin resistance, increased caloric intake during rapid growth spurts, and changes in hormone secretory patterns. After puberty, insulin requirements should decrease to $<1.0 \text{ U} \cdot \text{kg}^{-1} \cdot \text{day}^{-1}$ to prevent excessive weight gain. Dose requirements for pregnant patients vary with gestational duration and are discussed in PREGNANCY (page 94).

Most physicians start patients with newly diagnosed type I diabetes on human insulin. However, there is some concern about its relatively shorter duration of action, faster absorption, and possible tendency to produce more hypoglycemia in some patients. Careful balance of caloric intake, activity, and insulin dose are required for an insulin

regimen to be successful. If insulin dose is kept constant from day-to-day, food intake should also be kept constant.

The choice of insulin regimen should be based on individual characteristics, preferences, and habits, including age, stage of development, meal plans, and potential adherence to diabetes treatment. The health-care team should develop an acceptable and realistic treatment plan together with the patient. For example, an adolescent patient who is experiencing difficulties in following the treatment and presents frequent episodes of hyperglycemia or ketoacidosis may have to be treated with two injections per day administered by a family member or visiting nurse until his/her problems are resolved. Switching to less-frequent, longer-acting insulin injections ensures that at least the total insulin requirement is administered and may improve glucose control while avoiding ketoacidosis.

After the initial dose adjustments, ongoing long-term adjustments are made on the basis of daily repeated blood glucose measurements. Blood glucose levels should be monitored before meals, and at bedtime every day and on occasion between 0300 and 0400. With time and practice, patients and families are able to make the adjustments with relative ease and become progressively independent of the health-care team. In addition to the long-term adjustments, insulin doses and waiting times could be adjusted in response to high or low blood glucose levels, changes in food intake, activity level, or intercurrent illness. These adjustments can be made by patients who have been thoroughly trained and who can measure their blood glucose levels precisely.

Patient education is time consuming and should be conducted by a skilled health-care team working together with the patient and his/her family. It usually requires an initial period of instruction of 10–12 h, with periodic review and follow-up sessions every few months until the patient and family feel comfortable with their knowledge. Insulin regimens and blood glucose targets should also vary depending on the individual patient and should take into consideration the frequency and adherence to SMBG, the patient's ability to recognize and respond to hypoglycemic reactions, and the limitations imposed by what the patient and/or family are willing or ready to do. However, these should not prevent continued efforts toward the goal of achieving near-normoglycemia while avoiding severe hypoglycemia.

A frequent problem in the management of diabetes is the disappointment that sets in at the end of the honeymoon period when patients and parents of children with type I diabetes realize that the efforts invested in the treatment are not rewarded by the achievement of normoglycemia. Often, minor deviations from treatment or even no deviations at all result in unexplained fluctuations of the blood glucose levels. Because these fluctuations are part of the nature of type I diabetes, even under the strictest treatment conditions, such as with the use of multiple injections and insulin pumps, it is helpful at diagnosis to warn patients and families that the treatment of diabetes is imperfect and that blood glucose fluctuations are to be expected. Adequate explanations about the unpredictability of blood glucose levels and their relationship to daily variations of insulin absorption, food composition and absorption, and changes in the level of physical activity often help to prevent the development of feelings of guilt and incompetence that can plague patients and families. A useful attitude on the part of the health-care team is to stress the importance of overall blood glucose control rather than individual values, allowing for relatively wide fluctuations (70–160 mg/dl [3.9–8.9 mM] preprandial and up to 200 mg/dl [11.1 mM] postprandial).

INSULIN REGIMENS

General Principles

Normal insulin secretion is characterized by continuous basal release, with superimposed bursts of additional insulin inte-grated precisely to the rise in blood glucose after food intake. Additionally, insulin is secreted into the portal vein and thus goes to the liver before entering the general circulation. Ideally, exogenous insulin treatment regimens should mimic all aspects of this pattern. Unfortunately, with the available means of treatment, this is not clinically possible. Therefore, insulin treatment regimens represent varying degrees of compromise to achieve near-normalization of blood glucose levels, one of the most important goals of diabetes management. Ideally, insulin regimens should have both components of the normal insulin secretion.

Preprandial insulin is best mimicked by administering regular insulin before meals at the appropriate time, depending on the blood glucose level. Preprandial insulin comprises ~40–50% of the total daily dose.

Basal insulin secretion comprises ~40–50% of the total daily dose. It can be mimicked by intermediate-acting insulin given twice-daily at breakfast and supper or at breakfast and bedtime. The intermediate-acting insulins have onset of action after 2 h of the injection and produce peak levels 8–10 h after injection. Daytime NPH provides basal insulinemia. Bedtime NPH provides overnight basal insulinemia with peak serum insulins at around breakfast time and thus reduces the risk of nocturnal hypoglycemia. Long-acting insulin (ultralente) is given once daily before breakfast or at bedtime or twice daily at breakfast and bedtime. The latter schedule is relatively peakless after a steady state has been achieved. Its action could be sustained for up to 24 h.

Once-Daily Regimen

Among some adolescents and a few adults, a once-daily regimen, which usually results in only a minimal level of treatment, may be the only outcome achievable without alienating the patient. Once-daily regimens are sometimes effective for short periods during the honeymoon phase, when residual insulin secretion is substantial.

Figure 3.1. Various Insulin-Delivery Schemes (Before Individualizing for Meal Plan, Exercise, and Lifestyle)

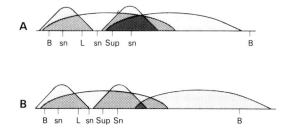

A

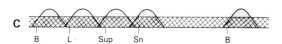

B

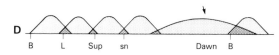

C

D

A: standard twice-daily insulin regimen (e.g., intermediate and short-acting). B: 3-times-daily insulin regimen, suggested for patients with early-morning hypoglycemia followed by rebound hyperglycemia or for patients with early-morning hyperglycemia (dawn phenomenon). C: multidose insulin regimen; 4 injections/day (short-acting insulin before meals and long-acting at bedtime). D: alternative multidose regimen consisting of 5 injections (short-acting insulin premeal and intermediate-acting insulin at bedtime). *Shaded areas* illustrate overlap between insulin peaks.

tion regimens commonly experience afternoon or evening hypoglycemia often in combination with nocturnal hyperglycemia. Frequently, a major improvement in glycemic control will result from a change to one of the two-injection regimens described below.

Whether such a regimen is adopted at the request of the patient or because the physician believes that patients will not accept more than one injection a day, it is almost always inadequate. Clinical and biochemical goals should always be reviewed with these patients, and sometimes a better understanding of the reasons for changing to more than a single morning injection leads to acceptance (see PHILOSOPHY AND GOALS, pages 17–18).

Twice-Daily Regimen

The morning short-acting insulin has major action between breakfast and lunch, and the intermediate-acting has major action between breakfast and supper (Figure 3.1). The evening short-acting insulin has major action between supper and bedtime, and its effect is reflected in the bedtime tests. The evening NPH or lente insulin has its major action overnight, and its effect is reflected in the blood glucose level on arising the next morning. The initial dose can be divided into 2/3 NPH and 1/3 regular at breakfast plus 1/2 NPH with 1/2 regular at supper. In younger children, the proportions are closer to 80%/20% for both components. The theoretical advantages of this regimen are *1)* the reduction of basal and postprandial hyperglycemia, and *2)* the reduction of overnight and fasting glycemia. The most frequent and serious disadvantage of this regimen is that in some patients attempts to achieve fasting normoglycemia result in nocturnal hypoglycemia (from 2400 to 0800) and early morning hyperglycemia (from 0400 to 0800, known as the "dawn phenomenon"). In these cases, it is better to move the intermediate-acting insulin to bedtime and thus reduce the peak effect of insulin from 0200 to 0400 and increase it at dawn. A representative case is

Although not usually recommended, this regimen uses a single morning injection of intermediate- or long-acting insulin, alone or in combination with short-acting insulin. The short-acting insulin has major action between breakfast and early afternoon, and its effect is reflected in the noon and presupper blood glucose levels. The NPH insulin has major action between supper and nighttime, and its effect is reflected in the bedtime and fasting glucose values. A helpful strategy is to start with 3/4 of the total dose as NPH and 1/4 as regular in young patients and 2/3 NPH with 1/3 regular in adults. An extra dose of short-acting insulin may be given before supper if blood glucose values are above the target. Patients on once-daily injec-

shown in Table 3.3. Generally, it is not possible to achieve near-euglycemia with two injections per day.

More Than Twice-Daily Regimens

Basal insulin requirements using either NPH or ultralente insulin with multidose insulin or basal regular insulin with continuous subcutaneous insulin infusion (CSII) account for ~50% of the patient's previous total daily dose. The remaining 50% is given as short-acting insulin delivered just before meals and/or snacks either by syringe, through an in situ catheter or pressure injector, or by an insulin pump pulse. A typical starting distribution would be 25% of the total daily dose as a short-acting insulin pulse to cover breakfast, 10% to cover lunch, and 20% to cover supper.

Alternative insulin delivery regimens of increasing sophistication include the following:

■ **Three injections a day** is a common variation if a two-injection regimen (with mixed doses before breakfast and supper) fails to deliver sufficient insulin to prevent fasting hyperglycemia. Typically, the 1700–1800 h dose of short-acting insulin is retained to counterbalance the glycemic effects of the evening meal, but the intermediate portion of that injection is delayed until bedtime (Figure 3.1B).

■ **Multiple injections** features injections of regular insulin preceding meals coupled with longer-acting preparations that mimic basal-insulin secretion. The regimen may consist of premeal regular insulin plus ultralente. The latter can be given once a day, before breakfast or at bedtime, or twice a day at both breakfast and bedtime. Another alternative is the combination of premeal regular insulin at breakfast,

---

Table 3.3. Case Study: Patient Who Takes Evening Insulin at Supper With Morning Hypoglycemia

Eight-yr-old Janine weighs 22 kg and is on a split-mixed regimen of human insulin: 3 regular plus 12 NPH prebreakfast and 1 regular plus 3 NPH presupper. Recently, she has had several hypoglycemic convulsions between 0200 and 0330, despite increases in her bedtime snack. Sometimes, but not always, the convulsions occur after an afternoon soccer game. A blood glucose profile reveals the following:

Breakfast		Lunch			Snack		
B	A	B	A	Supper	B	0200	0400
108	248	81	165	84	219	36	52
188	312	242	118	97	145	78	42

Suggested treatment

Overnight hypoglycemia commonly results from middle-of-the-night peaking of NPH or lente insulin, sometimes superimposed on the effects of late-afternoon activity. Verify that adherence is not an issue and that Janine's bedtime snack is large enough to balance increased exercise.

Divide the presupper insulin dose to provide 1–2 U regular insulin alone before supper (unless blood glucose is controlled adequately by morning NPH plus afternoon activity). Give NPH alone at bedtime to delay peak effect toward 0700–0800 rather than 0100–0300. Reduce the next morning's regular insulin to 1–2 U, because bedtime NPH insulin will be available to counter the postbreakfast glycemic rise. Morning NPH insulin may be increased a few units occasionally as well, based on pre- and postsupper blood glucose.

Recheck middle-of-the-night values to ensure they are >70 mg/dl (>3.9 mM), and reemphasize the need for extra calories or less evening insulin on the days Janine plays soccer.

lunch and supper with NPH at bedtime (Figure 3.1, *C* and *D*).

The combination of premeal regular insulin with bedtime NPH is quite popular because *1)* it offers flexibility in meal size and timing, *2)* it is very easily understood by most patients because each period of the day has a well-defined insulin component, and *3)* the introduction of insulin pens has made it very convenient.

Infusion Devices

Pump devices for continuous insulin infusion employ continuous insulin administration to normalize blood glucose levels throughout the 24-h period. Because insulin delivery is continuous, it can more or less mimic normal insulin secretion. Infusion systems have been developed for ambulatory use, which can use the intravenous, peritoneal, or subcutaneous route of insulin administration. These relatively small and lightweight portable devices (insulin pumps) can be implanted subcutaneously or carried extracorporeally. The most widely used method is the continuous subcutaneous insulin infusion with a portable extracorporeal battery-driven pump.

There are now devices on the market, with different features such as alarms for low battery, pump runaway, and empty reservoir, variable basal rates, and preprogrammed boluses. This treatment is extremely effective in improving glucose control in patients with type I diabetes. However, it should be restricted to very motivated and mature patients because it requires a high degree of cooperation. Although it has been used in children, insulin pumps should be used with caution in the pediatric population because of its severe potential complications. The complications resulting from this therapy may be quite serious. For example, hypoglycemia, probably the most severe complication, could result in brain damage and even death.

CSII delivers basal short-acting insulin continuously and permits the patient to administer bursts of insulin before meals (and looks similar to Figure 3.1*C*). Before initiating CSII therapy, the patient must receive careful support and instructions by the health-care team. These must include *1)* accurate and frequent monitoring of capillary blood glucose at least before each meal and bedtime; *2)* safe blood glucose targets during the night and early morning (>80 mg/dl [>4.4 mM]) to avoid hypoglycemia, the most frequent complication of intensive therapy; *3)* strategies to reduce the risk of nocturnal hypoglycemia, which include increasing the target fasting blood glucose to 130–140 mg/dl (7.2–7.8 mM), decreasing the basal rate if 0300 blood glucose levels are <80 mg/dl (<4.4 mM), and daily measurements of blood glucose levels at bedtime followed by an extra snack if the values are ≤140 mg/dl (≤7.8 mM); *4)* meticulous care of the injection site with frequent changing of the catheter to avoid cellulitis; *5)* excellent understanding of the pump functioning with special emphasis on measures to avert ketoacidosis, e.g., checking for obstruction or leaks in catheters with subsequent change in the case of unexplained hyperglycemia and checking of insulin reservoir; *6)* 24-h phone availability by experienced medical personnel; and *7)* the constant presence of a relative or friend until the patient becomes familiar with the treatment.

The initial programming of the pump is based on the total daily dose on the previous regimen. Approximately 50% of the total dose is given as the basal rate, and the rest is divided between breakfast, lunch, dinner, and snacks. Preferably, the bedtime snack should not require a bolus unless there is marked hyperglycemia (240 mg/dl [13.3 mM]). The basal rate is adjusted every 2nd or 3rd day on the basis of the blood glucose levels at 0300–0400 and at 0700–0800 until the desired blood glucose target is obtained. Increments should be in the order of 10–15%. In the case of nocturnal hypoglycemia, decrements of the basal rate should be larger. Premeal boluses are adjusted on the basis of the next premeal blood glucose level. Patients exhibiting the dawn phenomenon may require increased basal rates in the early morning hours.

Even when a patient's initial commitment persists, the use of pumps may be associated with various problems. These include local abscess formation at catheter sites, pump breakdown and/or malfunction, and forgetting to refill syringes or to change batteries. Undetected air bubbles or occlusions in catheters may obstruct insulin delivery, with resulting hyperglycemia, ketonemia, and even diabetic ketoacidosis.

Although some of these difficulties have been partly or completely resolved by the introduction of more flexible infusion sets (which reduce local irritation) and by buffered insulin preparations (which minimize insulin crystallization and avoid catheter obstruction), the major disadvantage remains the inexorable need for persistent SMBG. This will only be overcome when the need for SMBG is eliminated by implantable glucose sensors and servofeedback with (external or internal) mechanical insulin delivery devices not currently available.

INTENSIFYING BLOOD GLUCOSE CONTROL

Physiologic insulin secretion in non-diabetic individuals involves *1)* meal-related increased insulin secretion (initiated by neural and gut factors before the hyperglycemic stimulus), which is responsible for tissue uptake and storage of nutrients; this is followed by a rapid return of insulin secretion to the baseline; and *2)* basal insulin secretion between meals and during the night to regulate amino acids and fatty acids in the fasting state to prevent excessive nocturnal gluconeogenesis. Ideally, only an artificial β-cell with continuous monitoring of glucose concentration and administration of short-acting insulin into the portal circulation can replicate the function of the normal pancreas. Initial goals of glycemic improvement include approaching normal blood glucose levels without excessive or severe hypoglycemia. Therefore, a goal for preprandial blood glucose levels may start at 150–200 mg/dl (8.3–11.1 mM) but will decrease gradually to 80–140 mg/dl (4.4–7.8 mM). Ideal normal pre-

meal values of 70–120 mg/dl (3.9–6.7 mM) with 1- to 2-h postprandial values of <180 mg/dl (<10.0 mM) and a return to middle-of-the-night values in the range of 70–120 mg/dl (3.9–6.7 mM) are difficult to maintain safely except under highly intensive regimens in carefully monitored patients.

In the Diabetes Control and Complications Trial (DCCT), the goals of intensive treatment were to reduce the HbA_{1c} to <6% and to maintain this difference for up to 10 yr. In the trial, 44% of patients achieved that goal at least once during the study. However, <5% maintained an average value in that range. In response to the DCCT results, the American Diabetes Association recommended that "patients should aim for the best level of glucose control they can achieve without placing themselves at undue risk for hypoglycemia or other hazards associated with tight control." Therapy must be individualized. If the resources are available and the patient is willing, reasonable outcomes include mean plasma glucose of 140–160 mg/dl (7.8–8.9 mM) and HbA_{1c} values ~6.5–7.5%. In the DCCT, mean HbA_{1c} values were ~0.5% higher in adolescents than in subjects recruited as adults.

The implications of the DCCT findings are that optimal treatment should be offered to all patients. That means a progression from twice-daily to thrice-daily or multiple injections or the insulin pump depending on the response to treatment and the patient's ability and willingness to comply. An exception could be made in children because they appear to be at lower risk for microvascular complications until puberty and at higher risk of hypoglycemia. Moreover, younger children may be at higher risk for neurologic impairment with severe recurrent hypoglycemia.

To achieve near-euglycemia, it is advisable to use algorithms for adjusting both the insulin dose and the timing of the meal. Insulin algorithms are protocols for adjusting the dose and timing of insulin and meals based on regularly monitored blood glucose levels. They also allow patients to adjust

Table 3.4. Evaluating Blood Glucose Control: Factors to Consider

- Increase frequency of self-monitoring of blood glucose (SMBG) for 2–3 days; patient should measure blood glucose 6–8 times/day (fasting, pre- and postprandial, and bedtime values). Blood glucose values 80–120 mg/dl (4.4–6.7 mM) (fasting) to 180 mg/dl (10.0 mM) (postprandial) may be considered ideal; repeated values <70 or >180 mg/dl (<3.9 or >10.0 mM) are generally considered unacceptable and require action.
- With patient, identify the probable cause of high or low blood glucose values. Consider the following:
  - Exercise: forgotten, "burst" after long inactivity, prolonged
  - Snacks: forgotten, concealed, omitted, too small or large
  - Meals: advanced or delayed, time between injection of short-acting insulin and meal, day-to-day consistency in meal timing and/or size
  - Emotional upset: forgotten, considered unimportant
  - Alcohol or drugs
  - Illness or infection
  - Technique of insulin injection: into exercising limb or hypertrophied tissue; variation in depth, ability to draw up correct dose, timing of intermediate-acting injection
  - Technique of SMBG: timing, pad covered, meter readable, expired strips
  - Insulin reactions: treatment of undocumented, overtreatment, hypoglycemic unawareness
  - Deliberate nonadherence to regimen: insulin omission to lose weight, snacking, emotional problem, or eating disorder
- Note recurring glycemic patterns. Factors such as the following may be operative:
  - Fasting hyperglycemia: single-injection regimen/dawn phenomenon, rebound hyperglycemia
  - Late-afternoon hypoglycemia: single-injection regimen
  - Overnight hypoglycemia: intermediate-acting insulin dose too large or injected too early
  - Erratic glycemic patterns may also result from overinsulinization, antibody binding of insulin, or gastrointestinal motility disorders
- Alter therapy appropriately (see Table 3.5).

insulin dose in relation to amount and composition of food and exercise. Although flexible, such regimens tend to place greater demands on both patient and physician than a fixed course of treatment. Tables 3.4 and 3.5 present an example of a step-by-step approach to improving and intensifying therapy. The efficacy of insulin algorithms is predicated on

- reasonable and consistent adherence to meal plans;
- regular timing and adjustment of insulin based on SMBG;
- timing of the meal after the insulin injection; and
- regular pattern of activity or exercise or willingness to make adjustments in insulin or diet for unscheduled exercise.

Algorithms may be used to correct for a given value or to adjust insulin dose in anticipation of any blood glucose–altering factors, e.g., increased carbohydrate intake, most intercurrent infections, or decreased physical activity.

Once fasting and premeal values are in line with mutually defined goals, postprandial and middle-of-the-night SMBG can be performed periodically to double-check glycemic excursions and to perfect the treatment regimen. The patient whose average blood glucose value improves but who has recurrent episodes of severe hypoglycemia is, by definition, still not in good control. SMBG is as important for detecting and avoiding hypoglycemia as for identifying hyperglycemia.

Timing of Meals

It is preferable to give the insulin injection 20–30 min before meals so that plasma insulin levels are optimal for glu-

Table 3.5. Steps to Intensifying Therapy

- Obtain baseline (2–7 days) blood glucose profiles, glycated hemoglobin, and fasting lipids as well as baseline ophthalmologic and renal parameters. If the glycated hemoglobin value does not correspond to the blood glucose values, be certain that the patient does not have a hemoglobinopathy that precludes accurate assessment of mean blood glucose long term.
- If patient is on 1-injection regimen and profiles indicate hyperglycemia, start split-mixed regimen.
- Adjust meals and snacks to optimize timing, calories, and source of carbohydrate.
- Instruct patient to perform self-monitoring of blood glucose (SMBG) 4 times daily (prebreakfast, prelunch, presupper, and bedtime) and to keep detailed written daily records. Verify accuracy of technique by direct observation.
- Instruct patient to identify probable cause of high or low glucose values (e.g., overeating, late meal, skipped snack, excess activity, illness).
- Schedule office visits more frequently (e.g., every 1–4 wk) for detailed discussion and review of SMBG results feedback from staff, and help with problem solving.
- Increase SMBG to include postprandial periods and several measurements during the night. Examine SMBG pattern for subtle asymptomatic hypoglycemia or nocturnal hypoglycemia (with or without subsequent posttreatment hyperglycemia) as well as waning prebreakfast insulin effect.
- Adjust short-acting insulin doses according to individually constructed algorithms. Adjust meal times according to blood glucose values. All doses must be individualized for each patient. Use postprandial SMBG to recheck algorithm efficacy for correcting high or low glucose values toward 100 mg/dl (5.6 mM).
- Change from twice-daily injections to 3- to 4-times daily insulin if target glycemic levels are not met.
- If goals remain unmet, verify that dietary and SMBG adherence and contact with staff are optimal. If these are problems, redefine objectives to improve adherence. Use of an insulin pump is contraindicated if poor adherence is documented.
- Consider alternative ways to improve treatment by delivering insulin via available devices, e.g., an insulin pump, injections without needles (jet injection devices), indwelling subcutaneous catheters, prefilled cartridge injectors.

cose disposal. Patients should be instructed to vary the waiting periods depending on measured blood glucose levels. For example, no waiting time is necessary if blood glucose level is <65 mg/dl (<3.6 mM). However, the patient should wait 20–30 min when blood glucose value is 65–150 mg/dl (3.6–8.3 mM), 35–45 min if blood glucose level is >150–200 mg/dl (>8.3–11.1 mM), and 50–60 min if it is >200 mg/dl (>11.1 mM).

Compensatory Adjustments of Insulin

In addition to using variable waiting times, the patient may need to increase the dose of regular insulin to compensate for hyperglycemia, that is, use a "sliding scale" approach. This approach may be more practical for school-age children and patients who may not have the extra time to prolong the waiting period before the meal, such as when they have to get ready for school or work early in the morning. However, the advantage of the waiting time approach is that it may minimize the risk of hypoglycemia 3–4 h after the injection as a result of avoiding the relative hyperinsulinemia seen with the use of larger insulin doses used in the sliding scale approach. Some older children may sometimes withhold a carbohydrate-containing part of their meal for 60–90 min to help correct for hypoglycemia.

Long-Term Adjustments

Adjustments of the insulin dose are made on the basis of SMBG measurements and are aimed at achieving target blood glucose values. Adjustments should be made with care to avoid hypoglycemia and overinsulinization. Dose adjustments should not surpass 1–3 U (decreases or increases) and should be made only when persistent high or low blood glucose levels occur at about the same time of the day and cannot be explained by changes in activity, food intake, timing of the injection, or other causes. Adjustments should be made ideally every 3–4 days until the desired blood glucose is achieved, with the exception of unexplained severe hypoglycemia when it is safer to decrease the respective insulin dose the next day.

There are different ways to achieve treatment goals. One could start by changing the evening dose to normalize the morning blood glucose level while avoiding 0100–0300 hypoglycemia or, alternatively, by adjusting the morning dose to correct the evening blood glucose level. Generally, the adequacy of the morning short-acting insulin is judged by the postbreakfast and/or prelunch blood glucose level. Likewise, the correctness of the evening short-acting insulin is judged by the postsupper or bedtime blood glucose level. The adequacy of the morning intermediate-acting insulin is judged by the midafternoon blood glucose level, whereas the evening dose of intermediate-acting insulin is judged by the blood glucose level in the early morning and prebreakfast (e.g., 0200 and 0700) measurements.

When adjusting the evening dose, it is important to monitor the 0100–0300 blood glucose level in addition to the fasting blood glucose. Ideally, this should be >60 mg/dl (>3.3 mM); for most people, this is the time of the nadir value. Note that, despite repeated adjustments of insulin dose, hyper- or hypoglycemia may still occur; therefore, it may be advisable to adjust the carbohydrate content of the respective meal. For example, if changes in both components of the prebreakfast dose can achieve afternoon normoglycemia at the expense of prelunch hypoglycemia, the carbohydrate content of the midmorning snack should be increased. Likewise, if increases in the evening dose of NPH necessary to achieve in fasting normoglycemia result in nocturnal hypoglycemia, the carbohydrate and/or protein content of the bedtime snack should be increased. It is preferable to perform the bedtime blood glucose test at least 1 h after the evening snack to prevent nocturnal hypoglycemia. Added protein at bedtime may help prevent hypoglycemia in the early morning by increasing nocturnal glucagon levels.

The health-care team can develop an algorithm for the patient from premeal blood glucose determinations. A change of 1–3 U of short-acting insulin is prescribed for every 40- to 50-mg/dl (2.2- to 2.8-mM) increment (or decrement) in blood glucose level from a defined blood glucose target. This typical 1- to 3-U change is modified for individual patients based on the total dosage each day and sensitivity to short-acting insulin. Timing algorithms are described on pages 44–45. Carbohydrate algorithms are also available, but their use is not as well established.

All of the possible treatment options should be individualized according to meal plan, exercise, and lifestyle requirements. SMBG should be used frequently to profile glycemic values and to adjust therapy. Additionally, it is paramount that all treatment goals be mutually agreed on by the patient and the health-care team. Intensive therapy with multiple insulin injections or insulin pumps must be approached with knowledge and caution. All forms of intensive therapy require very high degrees of commitment on the part of the patient, the family, and the health-care team. Exceptional dedication, knowledge, and time commitments are the rule. Demands of insulin pumps are particularly stringent, requiring even more rigorous adherence to SMBG and other aspects of management and careful coordination by a team of experienced professionals. Because of the complexity of this problem, patients who are intent on achieving optimal glycemic control are best managed with an experienced team that includes a nurse trained in diabetes control, an endocrinologist (or pediatric endocrinologist), dietitian, and psychosocial counselor.

Barriers to Adherence

Even with initial commitment to intensified insulin therapy from the patient and health-care team, problems can arise. Many patients and their families are eager to intensify therapy until they experience the physical, psychological, financial, and practical day-to-day burdens such as continued meal planning, the difficulty of multiple injections or wearing a pump, catheter changes for pump users, more frequent monitoring, and more frequent office visits. Frustration with persistently variable blood glucose levels despite devoted, even compulsive efforts ultimately forces some patients into nonadherence. Some patients do well for 3–6 mo and then slip back into less rigorous patterns of behavior and deteriorating blood glucose control. When the goals of the patient and the health-care team are not congruent, attempts at intensive insulin therapy are commonly doomed to failure.

Glycated hemoglobin determinations not consistent with SMBG reports should raise concern that the patient is misusing the SMBG equipment, using a faulty or uncalibrated meter, or not providing honest or accurate data. It is possible that psychological problems have been overlooked (e.g., intentionally omitted insulin doses or eating disorders).

LONG-TERM THERAPY: COMMON PROBLEMS

Problems with insulin therapy arise regardless of the insulin regimen. They must be addressed. Detecting and eliminating patterns of hypoglycemia and hyperglycemia are the cornerstone of caring for diabetic patients. This is as true for the individual with diabetes of several years' duration as for the newly diagnosed patient.

Recurrent moderate or severe hypoglycemic reactions signal the need for evaluation of the insulin regimen, eating patterns, and other lifestyle factors (e.g., alcohol). Exceptionally low glycated hemoglobin levels may identify patients at risk for moderate and/or severe hypoglycemia. Some patients have diminished symptoms of impending hypoglycemia and, thus, suffer from recurrent hypoglycemic reactions and/or hypoglycemic seizures. In patients with hypoglycemia unawareness, blood glucose targets must be increased.

Fasting hyperglycemia may occur in conjunction with high or low blood glucose values. If SMBG between 0200 and 0400 reveals nocturnal hypoglycemia, rebound hyperglycemia (Somogyi effect) may be operative, although blood glucose levels >200 mg/dl (>11.1 mM) usually do not occur unless food is given to treat hypoglycemia. In this case, a decrease in evening intermediate-acting insulin is needed. However, if no nocturnal hypoglycemia can be documented, inadequate insulin from 0400 to 0900 may be causative. This should be addressed with either an increase in presupper insulin or a change to a bedtime injection schedule.

Inconsistencies of food intake and/or activity, often associated with psychosocial factors, can be causes of unacceptable day-to-day glucose control and glycated hemoglobin levels. Other factors that may contribute to glycemic irregularities are listed in Table 3.4, and a representative case is described in Table 3.3. Other problems of insulin therapy, including changes in insulin absorption or sensitivity, surgery, hypoglycemia, and insulin allergy are discussed in subsequent parts of this chapter or in other chapters (see INDEX).

Once the sources of hypoglycemia and hyperglycemia have been eliminated, further efforts to tighten control may require more intensified insulin-delivery protocols than are achievable with fixed twice-daily regimens.

INSULIN ALLERGY

Allergic reactions to insulin are increasingly rare with the widespread use of purified pork and human insulins. However, patients of all ages, particularly those with known atopic diseases, may exhibit local or systemic allergy to human insulin itself, protamine in NPH, or the zinc used in the lente insulins.

Some allergic-type reactions may be transient or artifactual. Burning, itching, and hives at injection sites may result from improper injection technique (intradermal rather than subcutaneous injection or injection of cold insulin) or from localized allergic phenomena.

If symptoms do not resolve and the patient's injection technique is sound, a change from beef and pork insulins to pure pork or human insulin or from one brand or type to another may be in order. True anaphylaxis or severe asthma, although rare, occurs occasionally and should be treated according to well-established protocols (e.g., antihistamines, epinephrine). If changing insulin type does not result in improvement, antihistamines can be prescribed. If atopic phenomena continue or if systemic symptoms occur, consultation with a diabetologist is recommended for alternative appr_ ches, including insulin desensitization.

SPECIAL CONSIDERATIONS

Exercise

Because exercise is a normal component of everyday life, it should be encouraged in every diabetic patient (see also pages 67–72). In anticipation of exercise, however, it is necessary to increase caloric intake or decrease the insulin dose to avoid hypoglycemic reactions during or after exercise. Hypoglycemia under these circumstances results from increased utilization of glucose by the exercising muscle as well as increased absorption of insulin from the injection sites as a consequence of increased blood flow. Injecting parts of the body that will least likely be exercised may decrease slightly the risk of hypoglycemia; however, because exercise usually increases the blood flow throughout the body, this may not be such a helpful approach. In the case of prolonged exercise (lasting >1–2 h), it is better to reduce the insulin dose because hypoglycemia could occur several hours after exercise.

It is recommended that, in anticipation of short bursts of exercise, one carbohydrate exchange per every 30–45 min of moderate exercise may prevent hypoglycemia. For exercise anticipated to last >1 h, a decrease in the insulin dosage according to the intensity and duration of exercise may be effective in reducing the risk of hypoglycemia. Table 3.6 shows sample guidelines for treatment in anticipation of exercise.

For patients on one daily insulin dose, a decrease is recommended in the dose of regular insulin if exercise is done within 3 h of breakfast. A decrease in intermediate-acting insulin is recommended if the exercise is done in the afternoon or later. For patients on twice-daily doses, a decrease in regular insulin is recommended if exercise is done within 3 h of breakfast or lunch, and/or a decrease in the morning NPH for exercise occurring in the late morning or early afternoon, and/or a decrease in the evening NPH in anticipation of exercise occurring in the late afternoon or after supper.

Management During Acute Illnesses

The increased secretion of counterregulatory hormones and decreased activity even in the face of reduced caloric intake or vomiting may increase insulin requirements. Blood glucose and urinary ketones should be tested frequently (e.g., every 1–4 h or each time patient urinates). The physician should be contacted immediately for advice. The following guidelines based on whether the patient is able to take food or liquids by mouth are useful for managing a child during an illness.

An illness not accompanied by nausea or vomiting (e.g., minor infection or trauma requiring bed rest). If activity is normal, give the usual dose of NPH/lente plus extra regular insulin as needed according to the blood glucose levels or urine tests. If blood glucose level is >240 mg/dl (>13.3 mM), increase by 20% the morning dose of regular insulin before meals. If blood glucose level is >400 mg/dl (>22.2 mM), increase the dose by 30%. If urine ketones are also present in

Table 3.6. Adjustments for Anticipated Exercise

Once-daily regimen
- Morning exercise lasting >45 min:
  - Decrease regular insulin by 25% for mild-to-moderate activity
  - Decrease regular insulin by 35% for moderate activity
  - Decrease regular insulin by 50% for strenuous activity (athletes in training)
- Afternoon or evening exercise lasting >45 min:
  - Decrease NPH/lente by 15% for mild-to-moderate activity
  - Decrease NPH/lente by 20% for moderate activity
  - Decrease NPH/lente by 25% for stenuous activity (athletes in training)

Twice-daily regimen
- Morning exercise lasting >45 min: Decrease morning regular insulin as above
- Early afternoon exercise lasting >45 min: Decrease morning NPH insulin as above
- Evening exercise lasting >45 min: Decrease supper NPH and regular insulin as for once-daily insulin

More than twice-daily injections
- Premeal regular insulin can be decreased for exercise occurring postprandially (from 25–50% decrements depending on the intensity and duration)

- Bedtime or morning NPH or ultralente should be decreased only for very prolonged and intense exercise (tournaments, marathons, etc.) ocurring at any time of the day

Continuous subcutaneous insulin infusion
- Premeal boluses should be decreased as above for postprandial exercise
- For light exercise, the basal rate can be maintained
- For moderate or intense exercise, the basal rate should be discontinued for the duration of exercise taking into account that a moderate amount of subcutaneous insulin remaining in the infusion site (3–5 U) will be absorbed.

For unanticipated exercise
- Insulin doses cannot be modified, thus hypoglycemia can be prevented by extra food
  - Mild to moderate exercise = 1 fruit exchange every 30–45 min
  - Moderate exercise = 1 starch + 1 protein before exercise + 1 fruit every 30–45 min during exercise
  - Stenuous exercise = 2 starches + 1 protein before exercise + 1–2 fruit(s) every 30–45 min during exercise

moderate to large amounts, an additional 10% may be added to these recommendations.

If activity is reduced and the patient is confined to bed, the diet should be reduced by approximately one-third. The reduction in caloric intake compensates for the inactivity. The insulin adjustment is the same as for an illness without bed rest.

An illness accompanied by nausea, vomiting, or marked anorexia. The insulin dose must never be omitted, because this could lead to ketoacidosis. In patients who have residual insulin or in very young children, it may be advantageous to omit the NPH or lente insulin in the morning and switch to a more flexible multiple injection regimen using injections of regular insulin at breakfast, lunch, and supper determined with a sliding scale (in doses commensurate to the blood glucose tests and the presence or absence of ketonuria) plus NPH at bedtime (~25% of the total daily insulin dose). If the patient is well by 1200, two-thirds of the usual total daily dose of NPH is given together with regular insulin (one-injection regimen) or one-half of the morning dose of NPH for those on twice-daily injections. If the patient is not eating or drinking and blood glucose level at fasting is normal, the dose of NPH insulin may have to be reduced. Extra doses of regular insulin may be necessary every 4–6 h in the case of hyperglycemia.

The meal plan should be replaced by regular soft drinks, fruit juice, or sweetened tea, 2–4 oz/h for children and 4–6 oz/h for adults.

Vomiting that occurs after the administration of the usual morning dose of insulin. Sips of sugar-containing fluids should be given every 20–30 min to maintain blood glucose levels between 100 and 180 mg/dl (5.67 and 10.0 mM). If vomiting persists and blood glucose level falls <100 mg/dl (<5.6 mM), the patient may have to be taken to the hospital for intravenous glucose therapy. A subcutaneous injection of glucagon should be given at home before departing if the patient lives some distance from the hospital.

Whenever blood glucose level is >240 mg/dl (>13.3 mM) and there is moderate or large ketonuria, the physician should be advised immediately, because this could reflect ketoacidosis. Repeated vomiting lasting >4–6 h or accompanied by high fever, abdominal pain, severe headache, or drowsiness may require that the patient be evaluated by a physician to ascertain whether he or she has a serious infection, appendicitis, meningitis, or other condition requiring antibiotics, surgery, or intensive medical care in a hospital setting.

Treatment of Diabetes in Infants

Transient neonatal diabetes can occur in newborn infants. These babies usually suffer from severe intrauterine malnutrition and, therefore, are small for their gestational age. They are hypoinsulinemic, fail to release insulin in response to any of the standard segretogogues, and must be treated with exogenous insulin with doses up to $1–2$ U·kg^{-1}·24 h^{-1}.

Insulin requirements are best established by starting a continuous intravenous insulin infusion at rates that provide at least 0.5 U·kg^{-1}·24 h^{-1}. Insulin treatment is simplified by using diluted insulins (e.g., a solution containing 10 U/ml) so that inadvertent overdoses do not occur. It is very important to dilute the insulin with diluents received directly from the manufacturer or, alternatively, to have the diluted insulin prepared by the manufacturer. In most cases, β-cell function develops sometime between the age of 6–12 wk. It is thought that there is a delay in the development of normal β-cell growth and differentiation. These children commonly do well after the newborn period and do not appear to be at increased risk of developing type I diabetes at a later age. Islet cell antibodies are usually not present.

Type I diabetes can start in infancy or during the neonatal period. The treatment is similar to that described for the infant with neonatal hyperglycemia. Insulin requirements vary and care of these patients should be supervised by an experienced specialist. Infants usually respond fairly well to twice-daily regimens with minimal or no short-acting insulin required. One of the problems found in these usually malnourished infants is that, due to the poor amount of subcutaneous fat, insulin injections are inadvertently given intramuscularly, and therefore, the duration of action is relatively unpredictable. If that is the case, an extra dose of intermediate-acting insulin should be added.

Local Reactions

Lipoatrophy and hypertrophy at the site of injection are the most common local complications of insulin therapy. The exact cause and incidence are not known. However, it appears that both occur less frequently with the use of purified insulins. Lipoatrophy improves with the injection of purified insulin directly into the area. In cases of local hypertrophy, rotation of injection sites with avoidance of the hypertrophic sites is recommended.

Insulin Resistance

Insulin antibody titers should be assayed in any patient with unexplained severe insulin resistance, i.e., >2 U/kg body wt after correction of ketosis with intravenous insulin. Patients with insulin resistance due to high insulin antibodies sometimes improve with corticosteroid treatment. Apparent insulin resistance may also occur as the result of patient's not taking insulin as prescribed or due to the use of insulin that has precipitated or aggregated from excessive shaking or heating.

CONCLUSION

Type I diabetes is characterized by a progressive decline of insulin secretion until its disappearance 1–5 yr after diagnosis. Thus, people with type I diabetes are dependent on insulin to survive. Insulin therapy is the most important aspect of the treatment of type I diabetes. However, insulin administration should always be coupled with SMBG. In this way, insulin therapy can be adjusted safely and effectively and individualized to age, lifestyle, eating habits, state of health, and physical activity. Effective insulin therapy helps the patient avoid extreme metabolic crises such as hypo- and hyperglycemia and achieve good glycemic control most of the time.

BIBLIOGRAPHY

Hirsh IB, Farkas-Hirsch R, Skyler JS: Intensive insulin therapy for treatment of type I diabetes. *Diabetes Care* 12:1265–83, 1990

Santiago JV, White N, Pontius S: Diabetes in childhood and adolescence. In *International Textbook of Diabetes Mellitus.* Alberti KGMM, DeFronzo RA, Keen H, Zimmet P, Eds. Chichester, UK, Wiley, 1992, p. 1026–57

Schade DS, Santiago JV, Skyler JS, Rizza RA: *Intensive Insulin Therapy.* Amsterdam, Excerpta Med., 1983

Zinman B: Insulin regimens and strategies for IDDM. *Diabetes Care* 16 (Suppl. 3):24–28, 1993

Monitoring

INTRODUCTION

Monitoring, performed by patients and their health-care team, is an integral feature of diabetes care. Specifically, results of blood glucose monitoring are useful in preventing hypoglycemia and adjusting insulin, diet, and exercise so that target blood glucose levels are achieved. Additionally, testing for urine ketones provides an early warning sign of impending ketoacidosis.

PATIENT-PERFORMED MONITORING

Patients can manage their diabetes effectively and safely only if they are able to perform self-monitoring of blood glucose (SMBG) levels. In certain circumstances (infants, infirm, or incapacitated aged patients), monitoring may be performed by family members or healthcare providers.

Urine Testing

In the past, the mainstay of diabetes monitoring was urine glucose testing. This method has distinct limitations and, therefore, should not be encouraged. However, if after repeated explanations about its disadvantages the patient refuses to monitor blood glucose levels, urine glucose testing is better than no testing at all to prevent excessive hyperglycemia.

Urine testing remains the only practical way to detect ketones (acetone). Testing for ketonuria should be a regular feature of sick-day instructions and every time blood glucose levels are consistently >240 mg/dl (>13.3 mM). The presence of persistent, moderate, or large amounts of ketones in the urine should prompt patients to adjust insulin as recommended or seek assistance by calling their doctor or nurse.

Urine ketones are measured preferably with reagent strips. Care should be taken not to use out-of-date strips.

Self-Monitoring of Blood Glucose

The most direct method of testing in type I diabetes is SMBG. This method allows patients to determine their blood glucose levels anywhere (at home, school, work, or while hospitalized) and to adjust therapy on the basis of accurate and timely results.

To perform SMBG, a drop of blood is obtained from a fingertip by use of a sharp lancet, usually with the aid of an automatic spring-loaded puncturing device. The blood is then applied to a chemically impregnated strip, and after a specified time, the resulting color change can be quantitated in a meter or read visually by matching it to a reference color chart. Generally, strips are best measured with a meter rather than by visually estimating their color against a chart.

Many commercially available strips and meters have been evaluated and are reliable and accurate. Lists of SMBG products are found in *Buyer's Guide to Diabetes Supplies*, published annually in *Diabetes Forecast* and available through the American Diabetes Association. With appropriate education, most patients can perform the technique successfully. However, office reassessment of the patient's skills (including the use of a meter every 6–12 mo if the patient is using one) and the use of quality control techniques at home are essential. Patients should be encouraged to bring their meters to every office visit to assess their accuracy. Inaccurate measurements can be more dangerous than no measurements at all.

Frequency of SMBG

The frequency and timing of glucose monitoring should be dictated by the particular needs and goals of the patient. Two tests each day, before breakfast and dinner, usually provide sufficient information to help adjust insulin and diet in patients taking one or two injections a day. Additional tests before, during, and/or after exercise can help the patient avoid serious hypoglycemia (see EXERCISE, pages 70–71). Patients on three or four insulin injections a day or using an insulin pump should test at least three times a day, before breakfast, dinner, and bedtime (to avoid nocturnal hypoglycemia). Adding a test before lunch is particularly important for patients who aim for near-normal blood glucose levels and for any patient during illness or intense physical activity.

Typical testing times should include prebreakfast (fasting), prelunch, presupper, and bedtime every day. Patients who have asymptomatic nocturnal hypoglycemia should be advised to test their bedtime blood glucose 1–1.5 h after the evening snack, particularly during very active days. In addition, such patients should test their blood glucose at 0200–0400, 4-5 times/mo. Patients should vary testing times to learn about their blood glucose patterns over the entire day. For patients who are well stabilized on fixed doses of insulin, routine testing (4 times/day) 3 days/wk (including 1 weekend day) may be sufficient. Conversely, patients who are ill (Table 2.6, page 28) or whose usual schedule has changed require more frequent monitoring. Table 3.7 provides typical monitoring schedules depending on the intensity of glycemic control.

Adjusting Insulin Dose

With SMBG results, patients on a split-mixed regimen can make appropriate insulin adjustments (Table 3.8). Occasional unacceptably high or low fasting blood glucose can be treated by adjusting the morning dose of short-acting insulin.

If fasting glucose remains in a consistently unacceptable range over a period of days, the evening dose of intermediate-acting insulin should be adjusted.

A late afternoon blood glucose reading can help direct the predinner short-acting insulin and the morning intermediate-acting insulin, which should still be fully effective before dinner. A prebedtime blood glucose reading can help determine the presupper dose, timing of short-acting insulin, and the size of the bedtime snack and can occasionally indicate the need for a small short-acting insulin supplement. Patients should be encouraged to take notice of persistent glycemic patterns and to correct for them. The dose of long- or intermediate-acting insulin should not be altered because of one odd test result. If blood glucose is consistently <60 or >240 mg/dl (<3.3 or >13.3 mM) or there is persistent ketonuria, the patient should be advised to call the physician.

Pregnant women or other patients who are intensively treated (multiple daily injections or insulin pump regimens) with the goal of achieving near-normal glucose levels will need to perform SMBG more frequently (4–8 times daily) to adjust insulin injections and to avoid hypoglycemia. As with

Table 3.7. Suggested Schedules for Self-Monitoring of Blood Glucose

LEVEL OF TREATMENT	TIME				
	PREBREAKFAST	PRELUNCH	PREDINNER	BEDTIME	OTHER*
Minimal	X - - - - - - - - - - or - - - - - - - - - X				X

To guide 1 or 2 daily injections of insulin and avoid hypoglycemia. Frequent insulin adjustments not made.

Average	X		X - - - or - - - X		X

To guide 2 daily insulin injections with mixed intermediate and regular insulins. Insulin adjustments made on a more regular basis.

Intensive	X	X	X	X	X

To guide frequent adjustments of insulin, meals, and exercise when goal is near-normal glycemia. Therapy with at least 3 injections each day or insulin pump.

*More frequent tests should be performed on sick days and when ketonuria is present, with changes in exercise or meal pattern, on travel days, or when hypoglycemia is suspected or imminent. Intensively treated patients should perform an 0300 test on a weekly basis. They may also test 1.5- to 2-h postprandial levels to achieve specified goals.
X, time of monitoring.

Table 3.8. Insulin Adjustments for Twice-Daily Insulin Regimen

Evening dose
- Increase by 10% the dose of intermediate-acting insulin if the fasting blood glucose is above the target for 3 consecutive days. (This modification can be made with the provision that the 0100–0300 blood glucose level is >70 mg/dl [>3.9 mM].)
- Reduce by 15% the evening dose of intermediate-acting insulin if 0100–0700 and/or fasting blood glucose levels are <70 mg/dl (<3.9 mM).
- Increase by 10% the evening dose of regular insulin if blood glucose 2 h after supper is >180 mg/dl (>10 mM) for 3 consecutive days. (This modification can be made with the provision that blood glucose level is >120 mg/dl [>6.7 mM] after the bedtime snack.)
- The maneuvers should be repeated until blood glucose levels are within the target.

Morning dose
- Increase by 10% the prebreakfast dose of regular insulin if blood glucose is above the target at midmorning or before lunch for 3 consecutive days.
- Increase by 10% the prebreakfast dose of intermediate-acting insulin if blood glucose is above the target before supper for more than 3 consecutive days.
- Reduce by 15% the morning dose of short-acting insulin if blood glucose after breakfast or before lunch is <70 mg/dl (<3.9 mM).

other elements of diabetes management, the prescription for SMBG must be individualized.

Additional Information From SMBG
The value of SMBG is not limited to adjustments in insulin dose. Patients with suspected nocturnal hypoglycemia can check their blood glucose levels at 0300 without being hospitalized. SMBG is a valuable educational tool to help the patient differentiate between symptoms truly arising from hypoglycemia or hyperglycemia and those from other causes.

Common Causes of Errors
Despite the relative simplicity of SMBG, the information is not free of errors. The most common problems, independent of specific methodologies, include the use of an inadequate drop of blood on the strip, poor technique in removing blood from the strip, and inaccurate timing. Test strips that do not require wiping and meters with built-in timers can help with some of these problems. These problems stress the need to provide proper patient education and training in SMBG. Finally, some patients report their results inaccurately, perhaps to please their health-care team with the right results. The use of meters that automatically store glucose results in an electronic memory may simplify the recording and reporting of SMBG, and these results should be analyzed periodically during office visits. Patients should still be encouraged to produce a written record of their test results to detect patterns. Faxing data saves considerable amounts of time.

Additional Points to Ensure Successful SMBG
If the goal of SMBG is to improve glycemic control, the health-care team should ensure that the patient:
- receives the necessary psychosocial support and technical guidance,
- monitors frequently, at least before meals and bedtime,
- reads and reports tests accurately,
- reviews results of glycemic patterns with the health-care team, and
- responds to the results by making appropriate changes in the insulin regimen.

To support successful SMBG, there should be mutual efforts to maintain education, motivation, and adherence. Furthermore, it is essential for the health-care team to provide feedback by monitoring progress with the determination of HbA_{1c} levels every 3–4 mo. Results of monitoring should be recorded and reviewed by the health-care provider at each office visit. Results can also be phoned, mailed, or faxed between visits. Health-care professionals must provide appropriate feedback to the patient based on monitoring results.

PHYSICIAN-PERFORMED MONITORING

Because blood glucose levels can fluctuate widely in type I diabetes, sporadic testing in the physician's office is not sufficient as the sole means of monitoring. Intermittent testing does not reliably predict glucose levels at other times or the level of chronic glycemic control. Laboratory glucose determinations should be performed occasionally to validate the accuracy of patient-performed monitoring and meter accuracy.

Glycated Hemoglobin

The introduction of glycated hemoglobin (HbA_1 or HbA_{1c}) assays has revolutionized the ability to follow glucose control over time. When hemoglobin and other proteins are exposed to glucose, the glucose becomes attached to the protein in a slow, nonenzymatic, and concentration-dependent fashion. The concentration of glycated hemoglobin best reflects the mean blood glucose concentration over the preceding 6–10 wk.

This measurement is performed on a single tube of blood or with a finger stick capillary sample, and when correctly performed by a reliable laboratory, the test is unaffected by acute changes in 90 blood glucose; therefore, it can be performed at any time during the day.

Assay Methods
Glycated hemoglobin can be assayed with several methods that measure different components of the glycated product (e.g., total glycated hemoglobin). Depending on the method used, actual test results, including normal ranges, will vary, and results from different laboratories cannot be directly compared. Physicians must determine which assay is being used locally and the nondiabetic range for that assay. Additionally,

certain medical conditions, e.g., hemoglobinopathies, polycythemias, and anemias, may affect the results of some methods. Radioimmunoassay and affinity chromatography methods are usually not affected by hemoglobinopathies.

Utility
A properly performed glycated hemoglobin assay provides the best available index of chronic glucose levels. Other glycated protein molecules can be measured for this purpose (e.g., glycated albumin), but their role in clinical practice is less well established.

Glycated hemoglobin is invaluable in identifying patients who have relatively high, average, or near-normal levels of chronic glucose control. Discrepancies between the glycated hemoglobin level and the results of SMBG or urine glucose testing may indicate that the latter are either inaccurately performed or fabricated. A less likely possibility is that the patient has some form of hemoglobinopathy that is interfering with the glycated hemoglobin assay: sickle hemoglobin spuriously lowers results, whereas HbF may spuriously elevate glycated hemoglobin in some assays.

The measurement of glycated hemoglobin allows physician and patient to set objective goals for therapy and to measure the efficacy of changes in therapy. The usual frequency for performing this assay in type I diabetes should be three to four times each year.

CONCLUSION

The appropriate application of self-monitoring of blood glucose techniques provides the patient with type I diabetes the opportunity to adjust therapy safely and effectively. The type and frequency of monitoring must be individualized and will be dictated primarily by the patient's lifestyle and the intensity of insulin therapy. Glycated hemoglobin measurement provides an objective index of long-term glucose levels and can be used to determine efficacy of treatment.

BIBLIOGRAPHY

American Diabetes Association consensus statement: Self-monitoring of blood glucose. *Diabetes Care* 17:81–86, 1994

Schiffrin A, Suissa S: Predicting nocturnal hypoglycemia in patients with type I diabetes treated with continuous subcutaneous insulin infusion. *Am J Med* 82:1127–32, 1987

Shalwitz RA, Farkas-Hirsch R, White NH, Santiago JV: Prevalence and consequences of nocturnal hypoglycemia among conventionally treated children with diabetes mellitus. *J Pediatr* 116:685–89, 1990

Nutrition

INTRODUCTION

The critical importance of nutrition in treating diabetes is well established. However, patients claim that diet is the most difficult part of their treatment regimen, and physicians attribute poor glycemic control to a lack of dietary adherence. To maximize the effectiveness of diet as the cornerstone of diabetes management, nutrition therapy must be individualized to achieve specific metabolic goals, provide optimum nutrition, and accommodate personal lifestyles.

The overall goal of nutritional management for type I diabetes is to enable patients to attain blood glucose levels as near normal as possible by integrating exogenous insulin into their usual eating and activity patterns. Diabetes nutrition therapy is initiated with assessment of the individual's metabolic and lifestyle parameters, implemented with a patient self-management plan, and evaluated through nutrition-related outcomes such as blood glucose and lipid levels, blood pressure, renal status, and normal growth in children.

The effectiveness of nutrition therapy depends on the ability and willingness of the patient to implement the treatment plan. Patients and their families should actively participate in setting treatment goals, developing their nutrition self-management plan, and evaluating the plan through self-monitoring of blood glucose (SMBG).

The complexity of integrating nutrition and insulin therapies and the importance of diabetes self-management education require a coordinated team approach to care of individuals with type I diabetes. Registered dietitians have the expertise to design the nutrition intervention and to counsel patients on nutrition self-management. Patients with type I diabetes should be referred when diagnosed, then routinely consult with a registered dietitian as part of the continuing medical care of their diabetes. Follow-up may be appropriate every 3–6 mo for children and every 6–12 mo for adults.

NUTRITION RECOMMENDATIONS

The American Diabetes Association has underscored the importance of individualizing diabetes nutritional care. New nutritional recommendations depart from previous recommendations by not setting optimal levels for macronutrient intake but advising that carbohydrate, protein, and fat content be individualized to achieve desired metabolic outcomes (Table 3.9). The "ADA diet" as a formulated prescription of calorie and macronutrient composition has been supplanted by a dietary prescription based on nutrition assessment and treatment goals. Specific goals of diabetes nutrition therapy are

- Maintenance of as near-normal blood glucose levels as possible by balancing food intake with insulin and activity levels.
- Achievement of optimal serum lipid levels.
- Provision of adequate calories for maintaining or attaining reasonable weights for adults and normal growth and development rates for children and adolescents and to meet increased metabolic needs during pregnancy and lactation or recovery from catabolic illness.
- Prevention and treatment of the acute complications of insulin-treated diabetes such as hypoglycemia, short-term illnesses and exercise-related problems, and the

Table 3.9. Nutrition Recommendations: Historical Perspective

	DISTRIBUTION OF CALORIES		
YEAR	CARBOHYDRATE (%)	PROTEIN (%)	FAT (%)
Before 1921	Starvation diets		
1921	20	10	70
1950	40	20	40
1971	45	20	35
1986	50–60	12–20	30
1994	A	10–20	A, B

A, based on nutrition assessment; B, <10% saturated fat

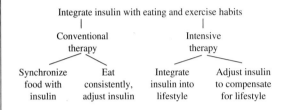

Integrate insulin with eating and exercise habits

| Conventional therapy | | Intensive therapy | |
| Synchronize food with insulin | Eat consistently, adjust insulin | Integrate insulin into lifestyle | Adjust insulin to compensate for lifestyle |

long-term complications of diabetes such as renal disease, autonomic neuropathy, hypertension, and cardiovascular disease.

■ Improvement of overall health through optimal nutrition. Dietary Guidelines for Americans and the Food Guide Pyramid summarize and illustrate nutritional guidelines and nutrient needs for all healthy Americans and can also be used by people with diabetes and their family members.

NUTRITION THERAPY FOR TYPE I DIABETES

Nutritional management of type I diabetes requires careful attention to the glycemic effect of food to contain postprandial blood glucose excursions, maximize the effectiveness of injected insulin, and minimize hypoglycemia. Nutritional care also must provide for optimal growth and development of the individual and reduce diet-related health risks. Although individuals with diabetes have the same nutritional needs as individuals without diabetes, the amount and type of food and timing of meals directly affects blood glucose levels.

Type I diabetes is easier to manage when people follow a consistent schedule and meals and insulin regimens can by synchronized to maximize glycemic control. Intensive diabetes treatment regimens, using multiple daily doses of insulin, offer greater flexibility in eating patterns than conventional therapy (Figure 3.2). Along with the type of insulin regimen, the nutrition treatment plan addresses caloric requirements,

macro- and micronutrient intake, the glycemic effect of foods and meal patterns, and lifestyle and lifespan modifiers.

Caloric Requirements

Calories should be prescribed to achieve and maintain reasonable body weight. Note that reasonable weight is defined as the weight an individual and health-care provider acknowledge as achievable and maintainable, both short and long term. This may not be the same as traditionally defined desirable or ideal body weight. Daily caloric requirements vary depending on age, sex, body size, and activity patterns. Additional calories are needed to promote growth during childhood, adolescence, pregnancy and lactation and for catabolic illnesses.

Several methods for estimating caloric requirements are available. Approaches that are fairly accurate, such as the Harris-Benedict or World Health Organization equations, compute calories for basal or resting energy expenditure (REE), then add activity calories to the basal requirement. A simple method for routine use is outlined in Table 3.10. Accurate records of food intake offer another means for estimating energy requirements and provide useful information on food preferences and eating patterns. Adjustments in caloric intake will need to be made to promote growth, weight gain, or weight loss. In addition to meeting energy requirements, the caloric prescription promotes a consistency in daily food intake that is important in managing type I diabetes.

Macronutrients

In general, recommendations for the macronutrient composition of the diet for diabetes correspond to guidelines for a healthy diet for all Americans. Emphasis is placed on an increased consumption of complex carbohydrate foods and a decrease in fat intake, particularly saturated fat. However, some lipid abnormalities, most often observed in non-insulin-dependent diabetes, may be exacerbated by a high carbohydrate

Table 3.10. Guidelines for Calculating Daily Calorie Requirements

AGE	CALORIE REQUIREMENTS
0–12 yr	1000 cal for 1st yr + 100 cal/yr over age 1 yr
12–15 yr	
Female	1500–2000 cal + 100 cal/yr over age 12 yr
Male	2000–2500 cal + 200 cal/yr over age 12 yr
15–20 yr	
Female	13–15 cal/lb (29–33 kcal/kg) DBW
Male	15–18 cal/lb (33–40 kcal/kg) DBW
Adults	
Physically active	14–16 cal/lb (31–35 kcal/kg) DBW
Moderately active	12–14 cal/lb (26–31 kcal/kg) DBW
Sedentary	10–12 cal/lb (22–26 kcal/kg) DBW
Sedentary, >55 yr, obese, and/or inactive	10 cal/lb (22 kcal/kg) DBW
Pregnancy	
1st trimester*	12–16 cal/lb (26–35 kcal/kg) DBW
2nd and 3rd trimesters	13–17 cal/lb (29–37 kcal/kg) DBW
Lactation	15–17 cal/lb (33–37 kcal/kg) DBW

DBW, desirable body weight

*2- to 4-lb weight gain; calories may be reduced slightly if obese, with early excessive weight gain, or with sedentary lifestyle.

---

intake and respond better to a diet with moderate levels of carbohydrate and less restriction in fat (see FAT below).

Protein. Protein intakes of 10–20% of calories are considered adequate to support health in the general population. Although dietary protein intake may influence glucose metabolism by altering gluconeogenic substrate and insulin and counterregulatory hormone secretion, there is not sufficient scientific evidence to support making recommendations for people with diabetes that differ from the general population. The Recommended Dietary Allowance (RDA) for protein is 0.8 $g \cdot kg^{-1} \cdot day^{-1}$ for adults, which corresponds to ~10% of calories. Protein requirements for children range from 2.2 $g \cdot kg^{-1} \cdot day^{-1}$ for infants to 0.9 $g \cdot kg^{-1} \cdot day^{-1}$ for adolescent males through 18 yr of age.

Data from animal models and limited clinical studies suggest that a reduction in protein intake is beneficial to treat, delay, or prevent diabetic nephropathy. The recent Modification of Diet in Renal Disease Study (MDRD), however, showed no significant effect from protein restriction on the rate of decline in glomerular filtration rate in subjects with varying degrees of renal insufficiency, although a small benefit was observed in patients with moderate renal disease. Individuals with diabetes requiring insulin were not included in the MDRD. A protein intake of 0.8 $g \cdot kg^{-1} \cdot day^{-1}$ (the adult RDA), or ~10% of calories, is sufficiently restrictive and recommended for individuals showing evidence of diabetic nephropathy. Evidence of protein undernutrition has been reported with protein intake of 0.6g $\cdot kg^{-1} \cdot day^{-1}$

Fat. The 80–90% of daily calories not allocated to dietary protein are distributed between carbohydrate and fat sources. The National Cholesterol Education Program (NCEP) recommends that all individuals over age 2 yr limit fat intake to <30% of calories, with saturated fat intake restricted to <10% of total calories. Saturated fat is highly atherogenic and has a greater impact on serum cholesterol than does dietary cholesterol. The NCEP recommends that polyunsaturated fat intake not exceed 10% of calories but allows flexibility in the area of monounsaturated fat consumption with a suggested range of 10–15% of calories. Dietary cholesterol intake should be <300 mg/day.

These recommendations are appropriate for most individuals with type I diabetes because *1*) diabetes is an independent risk factor for cardiovascular disease, and *2*) plasma lipid levels of individuals with controlled type I diabetes are similar to those of the general population of the same age and gender.

If individuals with type I diabetes have hyperlipidemia that is not associated with hyperglycemia, appropriate dietary modifications should be used. For example, if low-density lipoprotein (LDL) cholesterol levels are elevated, further restriction of saturated fat to 7% of total calories and dietary cholesterol to <200 mg/day is recommended.

Carbohydrate. A liberal intake of complex carbohydrates is recommended for all healthy Americans, including those with diabetes. Grains, vegetables, and other foods high in complex carbohydrates are good sources of vitamins, minerals, and dietary fiber. Traditionally, simple sugars, particularly sucrose, have been restricted in diets for individuals with diabetes. However, studies show that this restriction is not warranted metabolically. The glycemic effect of carbohydrate foods varies but cannot be predicted by their structure (i.e., starch vs. sugar) due to the efficiency of the human digestive tract in reducing complex carbon chains to monosaccharides. Studies to determine the glycemic potential of foods show that many factors, including processing, preparation, and meal composition, will vary postprandial glycemic excursions.

Clinically, the first priority should be given to the total amount of carbohydrate consumed rather than the source of carbohydrate. The amount of carbohydrate consumed at one time appears to be as valuable a predictor of glycemic excursion as any other parameter. For individuals with type I diabetes, the amount of carbohydrate in a meal, whether starch or sugar, should guide estimation of the amount of insulin needed to metabolize that meal. Carbohydrate counting is increasing in popularity as a diet planning strategy for individuals with type I diabetes.

Fiber. Dietary fiber appears to benefit overall bowel health, including prevention and treatment of constipation and possible prevention of colon cancer. Soluble fiber in large amounts (>20 g/day) has been shown to be effective in reducing total and LDL lipid levels in diabetic and nondiabetic subjects. The beneficial effect of soluble dietary fiber on glycemic control, although intuitively attractive, is difficult to substantiate.

An overall benefit to blood glucose control from dietary fiber has not been established and may require large amounts of soluble fiber supplementation to achieve a significant effect. Therefore, the current recommendation for individuals with diabetes is to follow the National Cancer Institute guideline for a 10–25 g/day intake of dietary fiber. The *Exchange Lists for Meal Planning* designate foods that provide ≥2–3 g fiber per serving.

Sweeteners. Sucrose restriction in the diet for diabetes can not be justified on the basis of its glycemic effect. As discussed above, studies show that the impact of carbohydrate foods on blood glucose is not related to compound structure. In fact, many starch foods (e.g., white bread, corn flakes) produce a greater rise in blood glucose levels than sucrose. Although glycemic effect does not differentiate starches and sugars, nutritional value does. Starches generally provide vitamins, minerals, and dietary fiber, whereas sucrose contributes "nutritionally empty" calories. For example, 8 oz regular Coke and 8 oz orange juice may not differ in their glycemic effect, but orange juice provides vitamin C along with other vitamins and minerals. Also, sucrose-containing foods are frequently high in fat, often saturated fat. Sucrose can be included in diets of people with diabetes by making appropriate substitutions so that the total carbohydrate content of the diet remains constant. Also, the potential for a decrease in nutrient value and increase in fat intake must be considered.

Dietary fructose has a low glycemic effect, which suggests that it could be the sweetener of choice for individuals with diabetes. Large amounts of fructose, however, can have an adverse effect on blood lipids. Also, many products are sweetened with high fructose corn syrup, which contains substantial amounts of glucose. Fructose provides 4 cal/g and in general does not offer strong advantages over other sweeteners.

Fruit juice, honey, molasses, corn syrup, and other natural sweeteners offer the same considerations as sucrose. They contribute 4 cal/g and need to be counted as carbohydrate in meal planning. Sugar alcohols (e.g., sorbitol) and hydrogenated starch hydrolysates have less of a glycemic effect than sucrose and possibly yield somewhat less than 4 cal/g. Some individuals report gastric discomfort after eating foods sweetened with these products, and consumption of large quantities may cause diarrhea.

Noncaloric sweeteners currently available in the United States include saccharin, acesulfame potassium, and aspartame. For tabletop use, noncaloric sweeteners in granulated form are packed with a bulking agent, usually dextrose, which contributes about 4 cal/packet. Several additional sweeteners are being evaluated by the Food and Drug Administration (FDA) and soon may be approved for use in the United States. The FDA determines an acceptable daily intake (ADI) for products it approves that is defined as a safe amount for daily consumption over a lifetime. The ADI includes a 100-fold safety factor and greatly exceeds average consumption levels. All FDA-approved sweeteners can be used by individuals with diabetes, including pregnant women.

Alcohol. With the exception of individuals whose blood glucose is out of control, those attempting weight loss, those with elevated blood triglycerides, and pregnant women, most adults with type I diabetes may drink alcohol in moderation if they so choose. Up to 2 servings a day (1 serving = 12 oz beer, 5 oz wine, or 1–1/2 oz distilled spirits) can be consumed with and in addition to the usual meal plan.

Along with the precautions regarding alcohol use that apply to the general public, people with type I diabetes risk alcohol-induced hypoglycemia when meals are skipped, delayed, or during fasting. Therefore, alcoholic beverages should be added to the meal plan without reducing food intake to balance calories derived from alcohol. However, if the patient is on a weight-loss regimen, calories from alcohol must be considered. Alcohol is best substituted for fat (1 serving = 2 fat exchanges).

Micronutrients

Sodium. People differ greatly in their sensitivity to sodium and its effect on blood pressure. Because sodium-sensitive individuals are not easily identified, intake recommendations range from no more than 3000 mg/day to no more than 2400 mg/day. For people with mild to moderate hypertension, ≤2400 mg/day sodium is recommended. Sodium intake can be minimized by reducing use of table salt, processed and convenience foods, and fast foods. The *Exchange Lists for Meal Planning* highlights foods with a sodium content >400 mg/serving.

Potassium. Individuals taking diuretics may experience a loss of potassium sufficient to warrant supplementation. Potassium restriction may be required if hyperkalemia occurs in patients with renal insufficiency or hyporeninemic hypoaldosteronism or those taking angiotension-converting–enzyme (ACE) inhibitors.

Vitamins and minerals. Although some research suggests an association between micronutrients and diabetes, at this time there is no evidence that vitamin and mineral requirements of individuals with type I diabetes are different from those of other healthy people. If a nutrition assessment reveals a deficiency, individuals should be counseled on how to adjust food intake to meet these needs. If they are unable to do so, supplements should be recommended. When caloric intake is <1200 cal/day, use of a multivitamin and mineral supplement should be advised. Several conditions may create a deficiency in one or more micronutrients that would warrant supplementation. These include poor diabetes control, use of diuretics, critical care environments, medications that alter micronutrient metabolism, strict vegetarian diets, pregnancy, and lactation.

ADDITIONAL NUTRITION CONSIDERATIONS

Sick-Day Management

Individuals with type I diabetes must be educated to manage brief periods when they cannot ingest solid foods. It is imperative for them to understand that some insulin must be continued and some carbohydrate consumed. Fruit juices and sugar-containing soda or gelatin can replace the usual carbohydrate in the meal plan. Frequent intermittent intake of small amounts of these foods and beverages helps to avoid hypoglycemia. Individuals should also be taught the importance of ingesting fluids containing sodium and potassium (e.g., vegetable and fruit juices and broths). The usual meal plan should be reintroduced gradually (see Table 2.6, page 28, for more on sick-day management).

Growth Years

For infants, children, and adolescents, height and weight data should be plotted on standardized growth grids. It is imperative that the caloric prescription for children with diabetes include adequate calories for growth and development. Poor diabetes control during the growth years can contribute to failure to attain height potential. During these years, it is helpful to schedule visits with the dietitian every 3–6 mo to adjust calories and other nutrients and to account for changes in food preferences and habits. Parents of infants and young children with diabetes may need more frequent nutrition counseling to deal with feeding problems common to young children but that present particular difficulty in type I patients.

Pregnancy

The 1989 RDA for pregnant women increases daily intakes of protein by 10 g/day and calories by 300 cal/day during the 2nd and 3rd trimester. A 1990 report from the National Academy of Sciences made recommendations for optimum weight gains for pregnant women based on prepregnancy body-mass index (Table 3.11). These guidelines anticipate delivery of babies weighing 3–4 kg at term. The 1990 report also stated that routine vitamin/mineral supplementation, other than elemental iron and folate, was not necessary during pregnancy. Folate given before conception and in early pregnancy reduces the risk of neural tube defects. Therefore, prescribing a multivitamin plus up to 400 mg/day folate from preconception through the 1st trimester is recommended. Assessment of nutritional status and dietary intake should guide prescription of supplements. Because of the additional metabolic stress of diabetes on pregnancy, nutritional guidelines need to be individualized for each pregnant diabetic patient to promote optimal blood glucose levels and maternal and fetal weight gains.

A plan of three meals and three to four snacks will help patients minimize blood glucose excursions and facilitate tight glycemic control. If there is morning ketosis with normal blood glucose levels, the amount of food in the prebedtime snack can be increased or a 0300 snack considered. In the 1st trimester, hyperemesis may be a problem. Insulin dosage should be adjusted to allow for minimum food intake at critical points during the day.

Lactation

The RDA for lactation is an additional 500 cal/day to include 15 g protein above prepregnancy requirements during the first 6 mo and 12 g/day thereafter. Many women with diabetes report wide swings in blood glucose levels while they are breastfeeding, which may be related to the amount of milk produced and the frequency of feedings. Continuing the pregnancy meal pattern of three meals and three to four snacks may help prevent hypoglycemia and decrease the need for additional insulin to cover the extra calories.

Obesity Management

Type I diabetic patients may gain excessive weight for several reasons: overinsulinization, overtreatment of insulin reactions, efforts to avoid insulin reactions with the use of extra food, failure to decrease caloric intake to compensate for decreased urinary caloric loss, and general emphasis on food intake. Parents and individuals with diabetes should be advised about the consequences of obesity on general health. Individuals with diabetes mellitus who are attempting to lose weight should avoid any fad diets that promote inappropriate food combinations and rapid weight loss, because dehydration, fluid and electrolyte imbalances, and starvation ketosis may result. Weight-loss programs for individuals with type I diabetes must include advice about insulin dose adjustment, careful monitoring of diabetes control, and realistic weight-loss goals.

Eating Disorders

An increasing number of children, adolescents, and adults in the general population appear to be affected with anorexia nervosa, bulimia, or a combination of the two. Type I diabetes mellitus complicated by an eating disorder is very difficult to manage because of erratic eating patterns and purging behaviors such as vomiting, laxative abuse, or excessive exercise. A purging behavior unique to type I diabetes is self-induced glycosuria, achieved by overeating with underinsulinization. If these destructive behaviors persist despite the expertise of the physician, referral to appropriate medical, psychological, and nutrition counselors is strongly urged.

THE PROCESS OF MEDICAL NUTRITION THERAPY

Medical nutrition therapy uses the same steps to patient care as other medical procedures. A patient assessment is used to determine treatment strategies, therapy is initiated and outcomes are used to evaluate effectiveness and to direct adjustments in treatment strategies. Although the dietitian is the primary provider of medical nutrition therapy, this component of diabetes management must be integrated into the care provided by all members of the treatment team.

Table 3.11. Recommended Weight Gain for Pregnant Women Based on Prepregnancy Body Mass Index (BMI)

WEIGHT-FOR-HEIGHT CATEGORY	RECOMMENDED WEIGHT GAIN	
	kg	lb
Low (BMI <19.8)	12.5–18	28–40
Normal (BMI 19.8–26)	11.5–16	25–35
High (BMI <26–29)	7.0–11.5	15–25
Obese (BMI >29)	≥6	≥15

BMI, wt(kg)/ht(m^2).
Adapted from Subcommittee on Nutritional Status and Weight Gain During Pregnancy, Food and Nutrition Board, National Academy of Science: *Nutrition During Pregnancy.* Washington, DC, Natl. Acad. Press, 1990

Assessment

Much of the information needed for the nutrition assessment (Table 3.12) is obtained for medical evaluation of the patient and is included in the education assessment (pages 22–23). Recognizing that the other members of the patient's health-care team need similar information should encourage communication among clinicians and collaboration on treatment goals.

Goal Setting

Specific goals for nutrition therapy are identified through the nutrition assessment. These goals must correspond with the overall treatment goals for the individual and must agree with the patient's personal goals for therapy. Goal setting is often a negotiation process involving clinicians and the patient. Goals should be realistic and specific.

Nutrition Treatment Plan

Modifications in the diet for type I diabetes are directed by the absolute insulin deficiency that characterizes the condition. Food intake and insulin regimens must be integrated to achieve maximum nutrient metabolism and avoid hyperglycemia and hypoglycemia. Fortunately, SMBG and multidose insulin regimens allow flexibility in nutrition

Table 3.12. Nutrition Assessment

CLINICAL DATA	DIETARY HISTORY	NUTRIENT INTAKE	SOCIAL HISTORY

Height and weight
Body frame
Reasonable weight
Blood pressure
Laboratory data
■ Blood glucose
  and lipids
■ Glycated
  hemoglobin
■ Abnormal laboratory findings
■ Insulin regimen
■ Family history
	Usual food intake
	Attitudes toward
	  nutrition and health
	Previous dietary
	  education and
	  outcomes
	Cultural food practices
		Overall nutritional
		  adequacy
		Caloric intake
		Nutrient distribution
		Type of carbohydrate,
		  protein, and fat
			Daily schedule
			Family relationships
			Friends—social support
			Finances and living
			  environment
			Education—learning
			  style

Adapted from Tinker LF, Heins JM, Holler HJ: see Bibliography.

planning to accommodate individual preferences and lifestyles. Specific strategies for nutritional management of type I diabetes are to
■ develop with the patient and family an individualized nutrition self-management plan that integrates insulin therapy and is appropriate for their lifestyle,
■ structure the meal plan to provide day-to-day consistency in caloric intake and in meal times and composition,
■ use information from SMBG to make adjustments in food intake or insulin dose to minimize blood glucose excursions, and
■ modify caloric and nutrient composition of the diet and meal plans as appropriate for different stages of the life cycle.

The individualized self-management plan should reflect the patient's lifestyle, exercise patterns, and insulin regimen. Important considerations are
■ daily schedule (weekday and weekend), travel to and from work or school, during work/school, recreational and social activities;
■ individual's and family's eating patterns including usual time and size of meals, food preferences, and social habits and cultural customs;
■ availability of food at home, school, or work; and
■ food budget, preparation, and storage.

Evaluation

The overall effectiveness of the nutrition treatment plan is evaluated by outcomes specifically related to the goals of therapy. Outcomes would include biophysical and lifestyle measures. SMBG provides patients and clinicians an evaluation mechanism that can be used to closely examine the effectiveness of the treatment regimen and make adjustments to improve glycemic control. Table 3.13 lists some options for meal by meal adjustments in food and or insulin dosages based on SMBG. Similar adjustments can be used to maintain glycemic control when alterations in the daily schedule affect exercise or food intake.

Nutrition Self-Management Tools

Meal planning tools, such as the *Exchange Lists for Meal Planning*, or the simplified version, *Healthy Food Choices*, can be used to guide patients in implementing their nutrition management plan. These tools are available from the American Diabetes Association, along with a professional guide on diabetes nutrition education and counseling. The Association also offers nutrition education materials directed to different

Table 3.13. Options for Regimen Adjustments Based on Self-Monitoring of Blood Glucose (SMBG)

SMBG VALUES	REGIMEN ADJUSTMENTS TO CONSIDER

Hyperglycemia

- ■ Fasting — Increase evening intermediate- or long-acting insulin dose or time injection later*
  - Decrease evening snack
- ■ Prelunch — Increase morning dose of short-acting insulin*
  - Alter breakfast meal plan by
    - Decreasing size
    - Adjusting composition†
    - Divide into meal and morning snack
- ■ Predinner — Increase dose of morning intermediate-acting or prelunch short-acting insulin*
  - Alter meal plan by
    - Decreasing or omitting afternoon snack
    - Decreasing size of lunch
    - Adjusting composition of lunch†
  - Increase activity level in afternoon
- ■ Bedtime — Increase dose of evening short-acting insulin*
  - Alter dinner meal plan by
    - Decreasing size
    - Adjusting composition†

Hypoglycemia

- ■ Fasting — Decrease evening intermediate- or long-acting insulin*
- ■ Prelunch — Decrease morning dose of short-acting insulin*
  - Alter meal plan by
    - Increasing size of breakfast
    - Adjusting composition of breakfast†
    - Adding midmorning snack
- ■ Predinner — Decrease morning dose of intermediate-acting or prelunch short-acting insulin*
  - Alter meal plan by
    - Increasing size of lunch
    - Adjusting composition of lunch†
    - Adding afternoon snack
  - Adjust time of lunch
- ■ Bedtime — Decrease evening short-acting insulin dose*
  - Alter meal plan by
    - Increasing size of dinner
    - Adjusting composition of dinner†
    - Increasing size of evening snack

*Options for insulin adjustments vary by regimens.
†Changes can be made in the amount or type of carbohydrate or the amount of protein or fat.
Adapted from Heins JM, Beebe CA: Nutritional management of diabetes mellitus. In *Management of Diabetes Mellitus: Perspectives of Care Across the Life Span.* Haire-Joshu D, Ed. St. Louis, MO, Mosby Year Book, 1992, p. 65

ethnic and regional food practices, several cookbooks, and a series of menu guides called the *Month of Meals* (see RESOURCES). A variety of new nutrition tools will be published in the near future. Additional nutrition resources that can be used effectively to treat type I diabetes are described in a monograph, *Meal Planning Approaches for Diabetes Management*, available from The American Dietetic Association (see BIBLIOGRAPHY). A meal planning tool should be selected that is appropriate for the patient's lifestyle, reading level, culture, and intensity of diabetes management.

Staged Nutrition Counseling

Eating habits are not easy to change. For the person with type I diabetes, the need to balance food intake and activity, the potential of hypoglycemia, and the psychological stress of managing a chronic disease make changing food habits even more difficult. Nutrition counseling should be provided in stages to allow the patient time to absorb information, try out self-management skills, and test the nutrition plan in daily living. Staged nutrition counseling also provides an opportunity to evaluate the effectiveness of the treatment plan and to make modifications to improve diabetes control. Nutrition therapy is a lifetime treatment of diabetes. Therefore, nutrition counseling must be included in the ongoing care of the patient with type I diabetes.

CONCLUSION

Diabetes nutrition therapy is more than calculation of a caloric prescription, with appropriate macronutrient composition and distribution of foods into meals and snacks. It is a complex process that requires much time on the part of clinicians and the patient to design an individualized nutrition self-management plan. The effectiveness of nutrition therapy is evaluated by success in achieving nutrition-related goals. If goals are not being achieved, the self-management plan needs to be adjusted either by modifying the amount and type of food at meals to improve glycemic response or by changing meal patterns to facilitate patient adherence. Nutrition therapy cannot be limited to the time of diagnosis, but must continue through life with adjustments made for growth and development, lifestyle changes, and for advances in the field of diabetes nutritional care.

BIBLIOGRAPHY

American Diabetes Association position statement: Nutrition recommendations and principles for people with diabetes mellitus. *Diabetes Care* 17:519–22, 1994

Daly A: Nutrition management. In *Therapy for Diabetes Mellitus and Related Disorders.* 2nd ed. Lebovitz HE, Ed. Alexandria, VA, Am. Diabetes Assoc., 1994, p. 95–101

Franz MJ, Horton ES, Bantle JP, Beebe CA, Brunzell JD, Coulston AM, Henry RR, Hoogwerf BJ, Stacpoole PW: Nutrition principles for the management of diabetes and related complications (technical review). *Diabetes Care* 17:490–519, 1994

Holler H, Green J (Eds.): *Meal Planning Approaches for Diabetes Management.* 2nd ed. Chicago, IL, Am. Dietetic Assoc., 1994

Powers M: *Handbook of Diabetes and Nutritional Management.* Rockville, MD, Aspen, 1987

Tinker LF, Heins JM, Holler HJ: Commentary and translation: 1994 nutrition recommendations for diabetes. *J Am Dietetic Assoc* 94:507–11, 1994

RESOURCES

Ethnic and Regional Food Practices. Alexandria, VA, Am. Diabetes Assoc., and Chicago IL, Am. Dietetic Assoc., various press dates

Exchange Lists for Meal Planning. Alexandria, VA, Am. Diabetes Assoc., and Chicago, IL, Am. Dietetic Assoc., 1989

Healthy Food Choices. Alexandria, VA, Am. Diabetes Assoc., and Chicago, IL, Am. Dietetic Assoc., 1986

Month of Meals series. Alexandria, VA, Am. Diabetes Assoc., various press dates

Nutritional Guide for Professionals: Diabetes Education and Meal Planning. Powers MA, Ed. Alexandria, VA, Am. Diabetes Assoc., and Chicago, IL, Am. Dietetic Assoc., 1988

Exercise

INTRODUCTION

In addition to insulin and a meal plan, exercise plays a key role in diabetes treatment; a specific exercise program should be an integral part of the treatment plan for patients with type I diabetes. Increased activity may help control weight, improve insulin sensitivity, bring about a healthier mental outlook, and reduce cardiovascular risk factors.

Given appropriate guidelines, people with diabetes can exercise safely. Children and adolescents can participate fully in gym classes, team sports, and other activities. Most adults should exercise more regularly and more vigorously. Disabled and incapacitated people can be taught how to exercise safely and should be encouraged to do so.

The exercise plan will vary for each patient depending on interest, age, general health, and level of physical fitness.

GLYCEMIC RESPONSE TO EXERCISE

Exercise requires rapid mobilization and redistribution of metabolic fuels to ensure an adequate energy supply for muscle contraction. In nondiabetic people, this complex process is coordinated via neural and hormonal responses that increase production of glucose and free fatty acids (FFA) and facilitate uptake and utilization of glucose by muscle (Table 3.14). In nondiabetic people, insulin levels fall while counterregulatory hormones rise, so increased glucose utilization of exercising muscle is matched precisely by increased glucose production from liver. In patients with type I diabetes, the glycemic response to exercise varies depending on overall diabetes control, plasma glucose and insulin levels at the start of exercise, intensity and duration of the exercise, previous food intake, and previous conditioning.

The important variable is the level of plasma insulin attained during and after exercise. Exercise increases blood flow and therefore the rate of insulin absorption from subcutaneous sites. Thus, although insulin levels in nondiabetic people will fall, in diabetic people they may rise. Excessive insulin levels can potentiate hypoglycemia because of insulin-enhanced muscle glucose uptake and inhibition of the rate of hepatic glucose production. The magnitude of the discrepancy between the rate of glucose use versus the rate of glucose production determines the timing and severity of hypoglycemia. In contrast, in a poorly controlled (underinsulinized) exerciser, insulin levels are too low, so that, with the rise in counterregulatory hormones during exercise, production of glucose and FFA continue, whereas uptake is minimal. This results in large increases in plasma glucose and ketone levels.

POTENTIAL BENEFITS OF EXERCISE

Clear-cut cardiovascular benefits accrue to patients who participate in a program of regular exercise. However, many other advantages, e.g., weight control and improved sense of well-being, can be achieved with even modest exercise programs that do not reach the intensity of exercise that improves aerobic capacity.

Physical training reduces risk factors for cardiovascular disease. Exercise is associated with a reduction in circulating levels of very-low-density lipoprotein and triglycerides and with an increase in high-density lipoprotein cholesterol, which is thought to protect against cardiovascular disease. In addition, exercise reduces blood pressure and increases cardiac work capacity.

When combined with a well-structured meal plan, regular exercise can make weight loss or weight maintenance much easier.

Physical activity increases insulin sensitivity. Glycated hemoglobin levels significantly improve with exercise only if the exercise is carefully integrated into a total-care program that includes meal plan adherence and frequent self-monitoring of blood glucose. Regular physical activity can ease the psychological stress often associated with a busy lifestyle. People who engage in regular

---

Table 3.14. Response to Exercise: Role of Insulin

In people without diabetes, insulin levels usually decrease during exercise, and glucose levels remain stable. In people with diabetes treated with insulin, insulin levels can increase, causing decreases in blood glucose levels.

People without diabetes

Utilization of glucose increases	Production of glucose and fatty acids increases
■ Glucose uptake by exercising muscle increases	■ Counterregulatory hormones increase glucose output by liver
■ Insulin decreases	■ Insulin decrease allows increased glucose release by liver and fatty acid mobilization

The result is precise integration of glucose utilization and production with stable blood glucose levels.

People with type I diabetes

Insulin excess: Occurs if increased blood flow during exercise increases (rather than decreases) plasma insulin levels; lack of suppression can also result in relative hyperinsulinemia.

Utilization of glucose increases	Increased production of glucose and free fatty acids is blunted
■ Glucose uptake by exercising muscle increases	■ Insulin excess reduces hepatic glucose release

The result is greater glucose utilization and reduced production, which result in hypoglycemia. This may occur immediately or hours after prolonged exercise.

Insulin deficiency: Occurs in poorly controlled (underinsulinized) patients.

Utilization of glucose by exercising muscle may be impaired	Production of glucose increases
	■ Counterregulatory hormones stimulate greater hepatic glucose release
	■ Ketone body production increased by increased counterregulatory hormones and low insulin

The result is a paradoxical increase in blood glucose and ketosis, which may progress to ketoacidosis.

exercise often experience an improved sense of well being; for them, exercise becomes an important and pleasurable part of their daily routine.

POTENTIAL RISKS OF EXERCISE

As with other medical therapies, exercise has risks as well as benefits.

Effect on Glycemic Control

Because prolonged and strenuous exercise can potentiate the effects of insulin, hypoglycemia during or after exercise is a definite risk for the individual with type I diabetes. In particular, it poses a risk for patients who exercise sporadically while continuing to take their usual insulin dose. Individual response patterns differ markedly. Some people regularly develop hypoglycemia during moderate exercise if no supplemental food is taken immediately before the activity, whereas others become hypoglycemic only many hours after the exercise. Because all patients with type I diabetes have some periods of relative insulin excess, it may be necessary to time the exercise so that it does not coincide with periods of peak insulin absorption or decrease the dose of insulin at work during exercise by one third to one half. Conversely, if diabetes is controlled at a minimal level or blood glucose is high before beginning activity, exercise may worsen metabolic control and increase ketosis.

Other Risk Factors

In patients with preexisting cardiovscular disease, exercise may precipitate arrhythmias, myocardial ischemia, or infarction. Risks related to underlying retinopathy and neuropathy and the inability to prevent hypoglycemia must be carefully considered. As in nondiabetic individuals, exercise can also aggravate preexisting joint disease or cause musculoskeletal injuries.

REDUCING EXERCISE RISKS

Potential hazards can be reduced if the exercise program is preceded by a medical evaluation, well supervised, and planned to progress gradually from low to more strenuous levels of exertion.

Preexercise Medical Evaluation

A preexercise medical evaluation should be performed regardless of the patient's age and should include:
■ assessment of glycemic control, including a glycated hemoglobin determination;
■ cardiovascular examination, including an ECG at rest and during exercise if the patient has indications of abnormal myocardial function;
■ neurologic and musculoskeletal examinations, including an examination of the feet; and
■ ophthalmologic examination.
  Exercise should be prescribed with caution in patients with frequent severe hyperglycemia or ketonuria; cardiovascular disease, neuropathy, or proliferative retinopathy; and hypoglycemia unawareness. These patients need to

choose types of exercise judiciously (Table 3.15) and consider increasing the frequency of blood glucose monitoring before, during, and after exercise.

Patients with known cardiovascular complications should have an exercise prescription developed as part of a cardiac rehabilitation program. Special precautions are also required in patients taking drugs that could mask the symptoms of hypoglycemia (e.g., β-blocking agents) or in people with other medical conditions such as hyperthyroidism or hypertension.

Instructions to Patients

All exercising patients should be given specific instructions regarding choice of exercise, glycemic control during exercise, and monitoring intensity of exercise. Patients should take appropriate safety measures (Table 3.16). The physician should review the risks of hypoglycemia and the dangers of exercise if diabetes is minimally controlled.

THE EXERCISE PRESCRIPTION

Exercise should be prescribed for the patient in much the same way as the meal plan and insulin. The key to success is individualization. The exercise program must be designed with the patient's input, taking into account age, lifestyle, level of physical conditioning,

---

Table 3.15. Precautions for Patients With Medical Complications

■ Insensitive feet or peripheral vascular insufficiency: avoid running; choose walking, cycling, swimming; emphasize proper footwear.

■ Untreated or recently treated proliferative retinopathy: avoid exercises associated with increased intra-abdominal pressure, eye trauma, Valsalva-like maneuvers, or rapid head movements.

■ Hypertension: avoid heavy lifting and Valsalva-like maneuvers; choose exercises that primarily involve the lower-extremity rather than upper-extremity muscle groups.

and motivation. Similarly, the duration, frequency, and intensity of exercise, as well as the type chosen, must be individualized. An informed exercise prescription is based on exercise testing that determines heart rate and blood pressure response to exercise and aerobic capacity ($VO_{2\,max}$).

An aerobic training program is desirable for almost everyone with diabetes. Some people may need to begin by first increasing normal daily activities (e.g., walking and climbing stairs).

Whenever possible, an "exercise contract" should be arranged with the patient. The agreed-on plan should be carefully documented and the patient's adherence to the program reviewed regularly and adjusted as needed. It is not enough just to tell patients that exercise is important and that they should do it regularly; few patients (or physicians) will respond positively to unstructured recommendations.

Aerobic Training

Patients who are interested and physically able should be encouraged to participate in aerobic training. Aerobic training stimulates cardiovascular fitness by using a large portion of the skeletal muscle mass for at least 20 min three times per week at a minimum of 50% $VO_{2\,max}$. Thus, a person who rides a stationary bicycle for 30 min but raises the work effort to only 40% of $VO_{2\,max}$ has not done much to improve cardiovascular fitness. This person would need to pedal faster, longer, and/or against greater resistance until heart rate and duration goals are achieved. Lifting light weights for many repetitions (high-volume resistance training) is an additional type of aerobic training.

If the clinician does not feel knowledgeable enough to personally prescribe and supervise an aerobic exercise program, the patient should be referred to one of the many programs available through physical education departments of local colleges, hospitals (particularly cardiac rehabilitation programs), and health and fitness clubs.

PREPARING FOR EXERCISE: ADJUSTING FOOD AND INSULIN

The meal plan and insulin dosage should be adjusted according to the patient's own response to physical activity. Because there can be major variability in responses, it is helpful for patients to monitor blood glucose levels before, during, and after exercise to learn their own response pattern. Generally, blood glucose values <100 mg/dl (<5.6 mM) indicate the need for a snack. Fasting blood glucose >250 mg/dl (>13.9 mM) with urine ketones or >300 mg/dl (>16.7 mM) regardless of ketosis requires insulin adjustment and delaying exercise until hyperglycemia improves and ketosis resolves.

Adjusting Food Intake

Moderate exercise of <30 min rarely requires any insulin adjustment, but often a small snack is needed just before the exercise, especially if blood glucose is <80 mg/dl (<4.4 mM). Longer periods of exercise almost always require snacks every 30–60 min.

Table 3.16. Guidelines for Safe Exercise

- Carry an identification card and wear a bracelet, necklace, or tag at all times that identifies them as having diabetes
- Avoid exercise during peak insulin action
- Consider reducing insulin dose when exercise is anticipated
- Administer insulin away from working limbs
- Be alert for signs of hypoglycemia during and for several hours after exercise
- Have immediate access to a source of readily absorbable carbohydrate (such as glucose tablets) to treat hypoglycemia
- Take sufficient fluids before, after, and if necessary, during exercise to prevent dehydration; and
- Measure fasting blood glucose and take appropriate action if
    <100 mg/dl (<5.6 mM): eat carbohydrate-containing snack before exercising
    >250 mg/dl (>13.9 mM): test urine ketones, delay exercising until ketones are negative
    >300 mg/dl (>16.7 mM): delay exercising until glucose is controlled

Experts differ in their recommendations for the type of food to be given. A serving of ~10–15 g of a rapidly absorbed carbohydrate for every 30 min of exercise is quite effective in preventing hypoglycemia. Examples include

- 1/2 cup low-fat ice cream
- 4 oz regular (nondiet) soft drink
- sports drink (consult label for amount)
- 1/2 bagel
- 3/4 cup Cheerios
- 1 small apple or peach.

The actual snack size required to prevent hypoglycemia must be determined on an individual basis and will vary depending on the duration and intensity of the activity. Patients who typically experience hypoglycemia only several hours after the exercise should take a snack after the exercise. For the patient who exercises in the evening, it is particularly important to monitor for nocturnal hypoglycemia and adjust the evening snack as appropriate.

Adjusting Insulin

Sometimes it is necessary to adjust the insulin dosage to prevent hypoglycemia. This occurs most often with strenuous activity of >45–60 min duration. The specific adjustment will depend on the patient's insulin dose regimen. For most patients, a modest decrease (~20%) in the insulin component corresponding to the period of exercise is sufficient to prevent hypoglycemia. If possible, patients should avoid injecting insulin in the extremity that will be predominantly used for the exercise.

For very prolonged vigorous exercise, such as prolonged running, backpacking, or long-distance cycling, a large decrease in the total daily insulin dosage (by as much as 1/3 to 1/2) may be necessary to prevent repeated hypoglycemic episodes. In this case, both short- and longer-acting insulin components may need to be decreased proportionally, depending on the timing of exercise in relation to the peaks of insulin action.

In contrast to these acute reductions in insulin dosage, individuals participating in long-term fitness programs often find that the total daily dosage of insulin will decrease by as much as 15–20%.

MONITORING INTENSITY OF EXERCISE

Regular participation in moderate or strenuous exercise is safer and can be quantitated more easily if patients know how to monitor exercise intensity by assessing heart rate, sense of fatigue using a rating of perceived exertion, and symptoms suggestive of myocardial ischemia. Patients can be taught how to monitor heart rate by palpating the carotid or radial pulse or by simply placing the hand on the left anterior chest wall.

The patient should take a 10-s count during the exercise or within 5 s of stopping and multiply the result by 6 to determine heart rate per minute. Patients should be alerted to stop exercising immediately if they experience chest discomfort or pain, severe shortness of breath, lightheadedness, or nausea.

Patients starting from a low level of fitness should also check their heart rate 5 and 10 min after the exercise session. It should be <120 and <100 beats/min, respectively. Shortness of breath should not be present after 5–7 min of rest.

Each session of moderate or strenuous exercise should include a warm-up and a cool-down period. Five to 10 min of stretching and flexibility exercises should be followed by more vigorous exercises, and the session should conclude with 10–20 min of less strenuous exercises and stretching. For the person who is poorly conditioned at the start, initial goals should always be very modest, starting with short (5–10 min) but frequent (5–7 days/wk) sessions.

CONCLUSION

Long recognized as a cornerstone of diabetes treatment, exercise is underutilized as a therapeutic modality; its hazards are too often perceived to outweigh its benefits. However, utilizing guidelines such as those supplied herein, physicians can frame a safe program of regular exercise that promotes the health and well-being of patients with type I diabetes.

BIBLIOGRAPHY

American Diabetes Association technical review: Exercise in individuals with insulin-dependent diabetes mellitus. *Diabetes Care.* In press

Campaigne BN, Lampman RM: *Exercise in the Clinical Management of Diabetes.* Champaign, IL, Human Kinetics, 1994

Fitness Book for People With Diabetes. Hornsby GH, Ed. Alexandria, VA, Am. Diabetes Assoc., 1994

Gordon NF: *Diabetes: Your Complete Exercise Guide.* Champaign, IL, Human Kinetics, 1993

Graham C, Lasko-McCarthey P: Exercise options for persons with diabetic complications. *Diabetes Educator* 16:212–20, 1990

Hough DO: Diabetes mellitus in sports. *Med Clin North Am* 78:423–37, 1994

Maynard T: Exercise. Pt. I. Physiological response to exercise in diabetes mellitus. *Diabetes Educator* 17: 196–206, 1991

Maynard T: Exercise. Pt II. Translating the exercise prescription. *Diabetes Educator* 17:384–95, 1991

Richter EA, Turcotte L, Hespel P, Kiens B: Metabolic responses to exercise: effects of endurance training and implications for diabetes. *Diabetes Care* 5:1767–76, 1992

Wallberg-Henriksson H, Wahren J: Effects of nutrition and diabetes mellitus on the regulation of metabolic fuels during exercise. *Am J Clin Nutr* 49(5 Suppl.):938–43, 1989

Special Problems

Highlights
Special Problems

DIABETIC KETOACIDOSIS

Diabetic ketoacidosis (DKA) is a life-threatening but reversible complication characterized by severe disturbances in protein, fat, and carbohydrate metabolism.

DKA is always due to insulin deficiency, either absolute (e.g., a previously undiagnosed patient or omitted insulin) or relative (e.g., too little insulin injected or antagonism by stress [counterregulatory] hormones).

Any major stress may precipitate DKA in a patient with diabetes who lacks sufficient circulating insulin.

The clinical signs and symptoms of DKA are listed in Table 4.1. They usually include polyuria, polydipsia, hyperventilation, dehydration, the fruity odor of ketones, and disturbances in the conscious state from drowsiness to frank coma.

The initial goal of therapy should be to correct life-threatening abnormalities, i.e.,
■ dehydration,
■ insulin deficiency, and
■ potassium deficiency.

Frequent reexamination of laboratory indices is imperative: at minimum, every hour during the first 4 h and at least every 4 h thereafter.

Routine bicarbonate administration is not recommended. Potassium administration is recommended for all patients. Some patients may require more aggressive therapy.

The cause of DKA must be aggressively pursued. Potential complications of therapy and how to avoid them are outlined on page 81.

DKA often can be prevented, given appropriate patient education and prompt physician attention.

HYPOGLYCEMIA

Hypoglycemia is a common side effect of insulin therapy. Mild hypoglycemic reactions usually consist of autonomic (neurogenic or adrenergic) symptoms, e.g., tremors, palpitations, sweating, and excessive hunger. Moderate and severe reactions include autonomic as well as neuroglycopenic symptoms, e.g., difficulty thinking, confusion, headache, slurred speech, dizziness, somnolence, seizures, or coma.

Mild hypoglycemic reactions may produce only minimal disruption of daily activities. Moderate and severe insulin reactions may severely harm health and morale and should be avoided.

Certain circumstances favor development of prolonged, incapacitating, and occasionally life-threatening hypoglycemia, i.e.,
■ hypoglycemia unawareness,
■ delayed treatment,
■ failure to notice symptoms because patient is sleeping or attention is elsewhere,
■ intensive glycemic control,
■ long duration of diabetes, or
■ certain medications or drugs.

The factors precipitating an episode of hypoglycemia can often be identified, allowing prevention of future reactions in similar circumstances (page 85).

Self-monitoring of blood glucose (SMBG) should be used to full advantage for detection and treatment of hypoglycemia. Changes in insulin injection, eating, or exercise schedules and travel call for increased frequency of monitoring.

Guidelines for treatment of mild, moderate, and severe reactions (pages 86–87) should be clearly understood by patient, family, and school and business associates.

Hypoglycemia may occasionally lead to rebound hyperglycemia, and should be recognized and appropriately treated if it occurs.

PREGNANCY

Women with type I diabetes who receive optimal care by an experienced health-care team can expect a pregnancy outcome similar to that of women who do not have diabetes.

Excellent glycemic control during pregnancy has been shown to bring unequivocally beneficial results to both mother and fetus.

Poor perinatal outcome is associated with poor glycemic control, ketonemia, and vasculopathy.

Patients should be as near to normoglycemia as possible at the time of conception and throughout the first trimester to decrease incidence of congenital malformations.

SMBG is mandatory during pregnancy.

Most women with type I diabetes may be managed as outpatients throughout gestation.

Tests to assess fetal growth and well-being should be conducted at appropriate times (Table 4.9). Timing of delivery and management during labor and delivery are covered on page 96. Postpartum care is covered on page 97. Family planning and contraception must be reviewed with the patient during the postpartum period.

SURGERY

Given appropriate preparation and management, patients with type I diabetes are subject to little more than normal risk during surgery.

Whenever possible, the patient should be in the best possible general health and glycemic control before a surgical procedure.

The objectives of glycemic management before, during, and after an operation are to prevent hypoglycemia and excessive hyperglycemia and ketoacidosis.

Because hypoglycemia is particularly dangerous, plasma glucose is generally kept between ~150 and 250 mg/dl (8.3–13.9 mM) during and after the operation.

Intravenous insulin delivery is preferred during surgery, although subcutaneous insulin may be used if the patient has stable glucose control, the procedure is relatively minor, and recovery is expected to be rapid.

In patients with DKA who need emergency surgery, efforts should be made to delay surgery until DKA is treated.

Guidelines are given for:
- major elective surgery (page 99)
- major emergency surgery (page 100), and
- surgery with local anesthesia (pages 100–102).

Diabetic Ketoacidosis

INTRODUCTION

Diabetic ketoacidosis (DKA) is a life-threatening but reversible complication characterized by severe disturbances in protein, fat, and carbohydrate metabolism that results from insulin deficiency. DKA is considered to be a medical emergency requiring treatment in a medical intensive care unit or equivalent setting.

In DKA, the arterial pH is <7.2, plasma bicarbonate is ≤15 meq/L, blood glucose is generally >250 mg/dl (>13.9 mM), and ketones are in the blood and urine. DKA is always due to insulin deficiency, either absolute or relative. It is absolute as the initial condition in a previously undiagnosed patient whose metabolic condition progresses to DKA or because a patient omitted a scheduled insulin injection. It is relative when too little insulin is administered or there is insufficient biologic activity of the insulin at the tissues because of the influence of counterregulatory hormones or other factors known to interfere with insulin action.

The counterregulatory or stress hormones comprise glucagon, catecholamines, cortisol, and growth hormone and are markedly elevated in DKA. Acting in concert, they antagonize the biologic effects of insulin and augment the metabolic derangements characteristic of DKA by promoting

- hyperglycemia secondary to increased glucose production and decreased utilization,
- osmotic diuresis and dehydration secondary to hyperglycemia,
- hyperlipidemia secondary to increased lipolysis,
- acidosis secondary to increased production and decreased utilization of acetoacetic acid and 3-β-hydroxybutyric acid derived from fatty acids, especially with dehydration and diminished renal blood flow, and
- an increased anion gap secondary to elevated ketoacids and lactate.

PRESENTATION OF DKA

The clinical diagnosis of DKA is usually apparent in a patient known to have type I diabetes. However, DKA may not be readily considered at first in an elderly, comatose patient with type II diabetes or in a child with new-onset diabetes whose rapid breathing is perceived as pneumonia. The diagnosis may also be confused with alcoholic ketoacidosis or starvation ketosis, because both conditions induce ketonemia and acidosis. A blood glucose concentration <250 mg/dl (<13.9 mM) usually excludes DKA unless the patient has been partially treated by additional insulin and fluids before presentation or has severely restricted calorie intake.

Clinical Signs and Symptoms

The clinical signs and symptoms of DKA usually include polyuria, polydipsia, hyperventilation, and dehydration (Table 4.1). The fruity odor of ketones will be apparent, and disturbances in conscious state vary from drowsiness to frank coma. Abdominal pain in association with an elevated white blood cell count and serum amylase may occur, particularly in young people, but it usually resolves with therapy. If severe abdominal pain persists, a surgical consultation should be obtained, because an acute condition such as appendicitis, bowel perforation, or infarction may exist.

Precipitating Factors

Any major stress may precipitate DKA in a diabetic patient who lacks sufficient circulating insulin. Infections such as pneumonia, meningitis, gastroenteritis, and influenza are some of the many heterogeneous causes as are trauma, myocardial infarction, and stroke. In most patients, it is possible to identify a specific precipitating cause. Among the most common are deliberate or inadvertent omission of insulin and mismanagement of sick days (withholding insulin from a patient who is vomiting and unable to eat, mistakenly believing it may provoke hypoglycemia) (Table 4.2).

ACUTE PATIENT CARE

The initial goal of therapy should be to correct life-threatening abnormalities, i.e., dehydration, insulin deficiency, and potassium deficiency. This must be done with great care. Fully correcting all biochemical abnormalities may take as long as 1 wk after the patient is eating solid foods.

Correct treatment of DKA is a feasible goal for all physicians. Frequent reexamination of laboratory indices is imperative to prevent serious electrolyte imbalance and fluid overload. During the first 12 h of therapy, the condition should be reevaluated at least hourly in the first 4 h and at least every 4 h thereafter. Particular attention should be paid to plasma potassium concentration. A flow sheet tabulating successive changes in the patient's condition must be maintained for all patients (Table 4.3). If the patient's clinical condition deteriorates after initial therapy has begun or if a metabolic complications occurs, consultation with an appropriate specialist is strongly recommended.

The degree of hyperglycemia, acidosis, dehydration, and conscious state is variable and depends partly on whether gluconeogenesis, lipolysis, or ketogenesis is the predominating metabolic abnormality. Other factors include the nutritional state of the patient, duration of DKA, concurrent drug therapy, and the degree of insulin deficiency. For a recommended treatment schedule, see Tables 4.4–4.6. Individual patients may require different schedules depending on clinical presentation.

Rehydration Process

Dehydration is present in almost all patients with DKA. There are many routes of water and/or electrolyte loss, including *1)* polyuria, *2)* hyperventilation, and *3)* vomiting and diarrhea. The

---

Table 4.1. Common Presenting Symptoms and Signs in Diabetic Ketoacidosis

SYMPTOMS	SIGNS
Nausea and vomiting	Tachycardia
Thirst and polyuria	Hypotension
Weakness and/or anorexia	Dehydration
Abdominal pain	Warm dry skin
Visual disturbances	Hyperpnea or
Somnolence	Kussmaul breathing
	Impaired consciousness and/or coma
	Weight loss
	Fruity odor of ketones

---

best index of the degree of dehydration is the magnitude of acute weight loss, which may be determined if the patient's baseline weight is known. Other clinical indices include orthostatic hypotension, dry mucous membranes, decreased tissue turgor, and thirst. A decrease in urine output is less reliable because of persistent osmotic diuresis with hyperglycemia. It is reasonable to assume an average weight loss of 5–10% of total body weight, or 3.5–7 L of fluid in a 70-kg patient.

Adequate rehydration is extremely important in initial therapy because it helps restore and maintain the depleted

---

Table 4.2. Points to Consider in Treating Diabetic Ketoacidosis

- A precipitating cause may be identified in 80% of patients.
- An ECG is indicated in all adult patients.
- Isotonic saline is initially preferred to rehydrate patients.
- Intravenous insulin is the preferred route of delivery.
- DKA patients are deplete in total-body potassium regardless of plasma potassium concentration.
- Bicarbonate is rarely needed; if indicated, do not give as bolus.
- Cautious replacement of phosphate is sometimes used.
- Preventing DKA is the long-term goal of good diabetes management.

Table 4.3. Ketoacidosis Flow Sheet

	MONITORING INTERVAL
Clinical*	
Mental status	1 h
Vital signs (T, P, R, BP)	1 h
ECG	As indicated
Weight	As indicated
Therapy†	
Fluid intake and output (ml/h)	1–4 h
Insulin (U/h)	1–4 h
Potassium (meq/h)	1–4 h
Glucose (g/h)	1–4 h
Bicarbonate and phosphate (meq/h)	1–4 h
Laboratory	
Glucose (bedside)	1 h
Potassium, pH	1–2 h
Sodium, chloride, bicarbonate	2–4 h
Phosphate, magnesium	4–6 h
BUN or creatinine	4–6 h
Urine ketones	2–4 h
Calcium	As indicated
Hematocrit	As indicated

Other considerations
Type and cross-match if necessary
Blood (and other) cultures if necessary
Aspirate stomach contents if comatose
Catheterize if needed for accurate urine output
   measurement
Give oxygen if indicated
Keep patient NPO

Therapy, laboratory data, and clinical assessment should be evaluated at presentation and monitored at frequent intervals for the 1st 12–24 h. In some assays, creatinine values are inaccurate with ketoacidosis.
*Patients with severe acidosis or hyperglycemia, hypotension, or mental status changes are generally best followed in an intensive care setting.
†Monitor every 1 h for 1st 4 h, every 2 h for next 8 h, and every 4–6 h, depending on response, for 24-h cycle.

vascular volume, and it enhances the kidney's ability to excrete glucose, thus lessening hyperglycemia. Isotonic saline (0.9%) is usually the initial choice of rehydrating fluid (Table 4.4). For patients who are hypertensive, hypernatremic, or at risk for congestive heart failure, a solution containing half (0.45%) isotonic saline may be preferable. In young children (≤10 yr), calculate according to body surface area, not weight (e.g., a 30-kg child has ~1 m² body surface area).

Insulin Replacement

Because the cause of DKA in all patients includes absolute or relative insulin deficiency, insulin must be provided. Although rehydration by itself will reduce plasma glucose, nonesterified fatty acids, and ketone bodies, insulin is required for suppression of ketoacid production and is thus necessary to correct acidosis. Insulin also inhibits glycogenolysis and gluconeogenesis, suppresses lipolysis, and facilitates the conservation of sodium and other electrolytes by the kidney.

Only short-acting (regular) insulin should be used initially. Replacing insulin intravenously is the most direct route and is preferred if methods are available to regulate the infusion rate. Replacement via the intramuscular route has also been successful, so choice will depend on the clinical situation (Table 4.5). Intravenous therapy may be started with a bolus dose of insulin (0.15 U/kg) followed by insulin infusion at a rate of $0.1 \text{ U·kg}^{-1}\text{·h}^{-1}$. This will bring about therapeutic insulin levels in almost all patients.

If no improvement in the acidosis as assessed by an increase in blood pH or bicarbonate or a decrease in the anion gap is apparent within 2–4 h, the infusion rate should be doubled. If this fails to ameliorate acidosis, the clinician should consider that more severe insulin resistance may be present. This might be precipitated by severe stress, e.g., myocardial infarction or sepsis, or by the presence of insulin antibodies in a patient who has been previously treated with insulin. Under these circumstances, consultation with a diabetologist should be sought.

Glucose is normalized more quickly than acidosis, and insulin infusion should be continued until both are corrected. Therefore, when blood glucose levels approach 300 mg/dl (16.7 mM), the insulin infusion should be continued but at a reduced rate (about half) while 5% dextrose is added to the infusion so that blood glucose levels can be maintained at ~250 mg/dl (13.9 mM) for the first 12–24 h. More rapid correction of hyperglycemia may increase the risk of cerebral edema.

Potassium Replacement

Patients with DKA are depleted in total body potassium despite a normal or even elevated serum potassium level. The reasons for this are complex and include the catabolic state, potassium wasting in urine secondary to polyuria, inability of the kidney to rapidly conserve potassium, and often, the effects of vomiting and/or diarrhea.

Correct potassium replacement requires both caution and timely action. The following procedure is recommended.

- Establish urine output to be certain the patient does not have renal failure.
- Send blood samples to the laboratory to measure serum potassium.
- Do an ECG to rapidly estimate if hypokalemia or hyperkalemia is present (high peaked T-waves in hyperkalemia; low T-waves with U-waves in hypokalemia).
- Begin potassium replacement at the suggested rate (Table 4.6).
- When laboratory reports are available, alter rate if necessary with the goal of maintaining the plasma potassium level between 3.5 and 6.0 meq/L at all times.

In most patients, once insulin infusion is begun, potassium replacement should be attended to promptly. Insulin tends to lower serum potassium by enhancing its movement back into cells. If potassium levels fall too low, hypokalemia-induced cardiac arrhythmia may result. Therefore, unless there is anuria, the clinician should begin potassium replacement within 1–2 h after starting insulin. If there is anuria, estimation by ECG lead II is not appropriate; replacement must await a plasma potassium determination by the laboratory, and potassium should be infused with special caution.

Table 4.4. Fluid Replacement

Hour 1
Provide 15–20 ml/kg isotonic NaCl (500 ml·m^{-2}·h^{-1}) or full-strength Ringer's lactate solution (if elderly patient or one with heart disease, administer fluid cautiously, e.g., according to central venous pressure).

Hour 2
Continue isotonic NaCl (15 ml/kg). However, if patient is hypernatremic, in congestive heart failure, or is a child, consider 0.5 isotonic sodium chloride.

Hour 3
Reduce fluid rate to 7.5 ml·kg^{-1}·h^{-1} in adults or 2–2.5 L·m^{-2}·24h^{-1} in children. Change fluid to 0.5 isotonic NaCl.

Hour 4
Adjust fluid rate to meet clinical need. Consider rate of urine output in fluid replacement calculation.

- When blood glucose approaches 300 mg/dl (16.7 mM), change fluid to 5% dextrose in 0.5 isotonic NaCl. Continue intravenous fluids, including insulin, until acidosis is corrected and patient can ingest food without vomiting. Then change to short-acting insulin subcutaneously every 4–6 h, giving first dose before discontinuing intravenous insulin.
- Many specialists recommend intermediate-acting insulin, before discontinuation of intravenous insulin, so that a depot of insulin is available. Supplemental short-acting insulin is added as necessary, guided by blood glucose concentration.

Additional potassium may be needed if the patient is receiving sodium bicarbonate, because bicarbonate further enhances hypokalemia by promoting potassium movement back into cells.

Bicarbonate and Phosphate Replacement

Although it seems reasonable to administer sodium bicarbonate to the patient with DKA to correct the metabolic acidosis with alkali, it is not clear whether the potential benefits outweigh potential risks. The potential benefits of administering sodium bicarbonate include

- correcting extracellular acidosis,
- reducing excessive chloride administration,
- reducing respiratory rate and increasing comfort,

Table 4.5. Insulin Administration: Initially Use Short-Acting (Regular) Insulin Only

Intravenous route preferred
- Bolus dose 0.15 U/kg
- Continuous infusion 0.1 $U \cdot kg^{-1} \cdot h^{-1}$ before connecting infusion tubing to patient, run 30 ml of insulin solution through tubing to saturate tubing absorption sites.
- Changing insulin infusion rate
  - If no biochemical response is detected by 2–4 h, then double infusion rate (be sure to first check all infusion lines for patency and that insulin was added to IV bottle).
  - If blood glucose declines <300 mg/dl (<16.7 mM), then halve the infusion rate of insulin or add 5% dextrose (do not stop insulin infusion).
- Discontinuing infusion
  - Inject subcutaneous insulin.
  - 30 min later, discontinue intravenous infusion.

Intramuscular route recommended only if no method is available to regulate intravenous insulin infusion rate
- First hour of therapy, 0.5 U/kg
- Each hour thereafter, 0.1 U/kg until blood glucose is reduced to 300 mg/dl (16.7 mM)
- Every 2 h thereafter, inject 0.1 U/kg as necessary to maintain blood glucose concentration at 250 mg/dl (13.9 mM). Some specialists recommend intermediate-acting insulin.

- reducing cardiac irritability, and
- increasing responsiveness of vascular system to pressor agents.

However, the potential harmful effects include
- accelerated reduction in plasma potassium concentration,
- sodium overload in elderly patients, and
- exacerbating intracellular acidosis.

For these reasons, routine bicarbonate administration is not recommended in most cases of DKA when pH is ≥7.1. Some authorities still recommend administration of bicarbonate in patients with severe acidosis (i.e., pH <7.0), particularly when hypotension, shock, and arrhythmias are also present. Bicarbonate should be given as an infusion of 1–2 meq/kg over 2 h, and then the plasma bicarbonate level should be checked. The amount of bicarbonate administered should generally not exceed 3 meq/kg over 12 h.

Patients presenting in DKA are usually phosphate depleted from a combination of decreased food intake, excessive catabolism, and increased urinary excretion. Furthermore, as with potassium, administering insulin enhances the movement of phosphate into cells, further reducing the plasma phosphate concentration.

There are pros and cons to administering phosphate, an ion important to many chemical reactions at the cellular level. One potential benefit is that hyperchloremia may be less likely to result when potassium is replaced as potassium phosphate instead of potassium chloride. However, administering too much phosphate can induce hypocalcemia. Therefore, calcium levels should be checked before phosphate is administered.

Although routine phosphate replacement has not been shown to be of benefit in the treatment of DKA, conservative potassium phosphate administration not to exceed 1.5 $meq \cdot kg^{-1} \cdot 24\ h^{-1}$ is usually recommended for all patients. In this way, most of the potassium is administered as potassium chloride. More aggressive phosphate therapy should be considered in patients with a low initial phosphate concentration (≤2 meq/L) or evidence of phosphate depletion syndrome, e.g., rhabdomyolysis.

OTHER IMPORTANT CONSIDERATIONS

It is important to pursue other aspects of therapy while correcting the laboratory abnormalities. First and foremost, the cause of DKA must be pursued aggressively in both previously and newly diagnosed patients. Even if omission of an insulin injection by the patient is documented, the physician must be certain that there is no coexisting medical condition. In several reported series of adult patients admitted to the hospital with DKA, infection was the most common precipitating factor. Therefore, depending on clinical signs and symptoms, a chest X ray plus culture of the urine, throat, sputum, and blood may be warranted. Antibiotics should be considered in all cases of suspected infection. In adult patients, an ECG is mandatory because myocardial infarction may be precipitate DKA. As previously discussed, the clinician should also carefully investigate all possible causes of abdominal pain.

In addition to determination of the cause of DKA, other supportive therapy must be considered. Ensuring an airway and inserting a nasogastric tube to drain gastric contents in comatose patients are strongly recommended to prevent aspiration pneumonia. Low-dose subcutaneous heparin (5000 U every 12 h) is often recommended to prevent hypercoagulability, especially in elderly patients. However, data that demonstrate the benefit of heparin administration in DKA are lacking.

Be alert to complications of treatment. Potential complications directly attributable to the treatment of DKA must be anticipated.

- Generally, glucose will be normalized more quickly than acidosis. Premature discontinuation of insulin may result in persistence and worsening of ketoacidosis.
- Cerebral edema and death may occur, particularly in children. Although the etiology of this complication has not been determined, some authorities believe that it is caused by correcting hyperglycemia too rapidly and the use of excessive amounts of hypotomic fluid. Therefore, the blood glucose concentration should be maintained at ~250 mg/dl (~13.9 mM) during the first 12–24 h.
- Nausea and vomiting from feeding the patient before gastric peristalsis has returned can result in aspiration pneumonia. Therefore, solid foods should be introduced cautiously.
- Hypoglycemia can occur if the insulin infusion is not supplemented with glucose when the blood glucose concentration is <300 mg/dl (<16.7 mM). If acidosis is still present, the insulin infusion must be continued at 0.05–0.1 U·kg^{-1}·h^{-1}, and glucose must be infused to maintain the blood glucose concentration >200 mg/dl (>11.1 mM).

Table 4.6. Potassium Replacement

- Initially, in patients with adequate urine output, ECG (lead II) may be used as a guide for plasma K$^+$ concentration.

- Replacement of K$^+$ is based on plasma K$^+$ concentration. If K$^+$ is
  - <3 meq/L, infuse ≥0.6 meq·kg^{-1}·h^{-1}
  - 3–4 meq/L, infuse 0.6 meq·kg^{-1}·h^{-1}
  - 4–5 meq/L, infuse 0.2–0.4 meq·kg^{-1}·h^{-1}
  - 5–6 meq/L, infuse 0.1–0.2 meq·kg^{-1}·h^{-1}
  - 6 meq/L, withhold until K$^+$ is <6.0 meq/L

- Add K$^+$ to replacement fluid therapy. If concentration of K$^+$ in infusate is 20–40 meq/L and infusion into peripheral vein causes irritation, infuse into central vein.

- Recheck plasma K$^+$ every 2 h if plasma concentration is <4 or >6 meq/L.

- Administer K$^+$ as K$^+$Cl$^-$ or as potassium phosphate. However, do not exceed 90 meq/24 h potassium phosphate because of danger of hypocalcemia.

- Use higher end of suggested range if bicarbonate is also being administered.

- Too aggressive fluid replacement (particularly with isotonic saline) may induce congestive heart failure. Therefore, frequent auscultation of the lungs is mandatory.

Intermediate Patient Care

As the patient improves, the question of when to discontinue intravenous insulin and fluids and begin subcutaneous insulin will arise. To answer this question, several clinical parameters must be considered:

- Is the patient clinically stable with normal vital signs?
- Has the patient's blood pH, plasma bicarbonate level, or anion gap returned toward normal levels (i.e., has the acidosis been corrected)?
- Can the patient drink fluids without experiencing nausea and vomiting?
- Has the precipitating stress (e.g., infection) been controlled?

If the answer to any of these questions is no, then the physician should probably continue intravenous insulin and fluid.

When subcutaneous insulin is begun, three points should be considered. First, because subcutaneous insulin takes effect more slowly than intravenous insulin loses its effectiveness, the first subcutaneous insulin injection should be given at least 15–30 min before termination of the intravenous insulin infusion. This initial dose should be ~0.2 U/kg, and blood glucose should be checked every 4–6 h to determine whether an increase or a decrease in insulin is needed. Second, some clinicians prefer to use short-acting insulin only, in divided doses (0.1–0.25 U/kg) every 4–6 h for the first 24 h, before beginning a regimen with a longer-acting insulin such as NPH or lente. Short-acting insulin permits rapid adjustment of the insulin dose to control blood glucose during this transition phase. Other authorities recommended the use of intermediate-acting insulin (0.2 U/kg) from the outset to prevent recurrence of acidosis in the transition phase. If the patient was receiving insulin previously, the prior dose should be used as a guide to reinstituting therapy. Third, the patient may remain mildly insulin resistant for several weeks, so the dose of subcutaneous insulin may exceed the patient's usual requirements.

PREVENTIVE CARE

Most often, DKA can be prevented, given appropriate patient education and prompt physician attention. All patients with diabetes should know how to perform self-monitoring of blood glucose (SMBG) and urine ketone testing. Patients must learn to contact their physicians as soon as they become ill, have nausea and vomiting, fever, or persistent hyperglycemia or hyperketonuria. When contacted early, the physician is often able to treat DKA successfully by prescribing frequent injections of short-acting insulin and by oral administration of fluids. It may also be possible to rehydrate and reinsulinize the patient in the doctor's office or emergency room, thereby preventing progression to DKA and expensive hospitalization.

However, when there is any doubt that the patient can be successfully treated in the emergency room, hospitalization is indicated. For patients who have repeated episodes of DKA, psychological consultation should be considered. Many of these patients, especially adolescents, may use the hospital as a haven from social and psychological pressures.

CONCLUSION

The pathophysiology of DKA can now be understood in the context of insulin deficiency and excessive counterregulatory hormones combining their effects to produce a severe state of life-threatening metabolic decompensation. Insulin, fluids, and electrolytes, given judiciously under appropriate guidelines in a hospital setting, form the cornerstone of treatment. A precipitating event such as infection, infarction, or deliberate omission of insulin must be identified and treated.

BIBLIOGRAPHY

Bratton SL, Krane EJ: Diabetic ketoacidosis: pathophysiology, management, and complications. *Intensive Care Med* 7:199–211, 1992

DeFronzo RA, Matsuda M, Barrett EJ: Diabetic ketoacidosis: a combined metabolic-nephrologic approach to therapy. *Diabetes Rev* 2:209–38, 1994

Kaufman FR: Treatment strategies for diabetic ketoacidosis in children and adolescents with insulin-dependent diabetes mellitus. *Clin Diabetes* 11:102–106, 1993

Marshall SM, Walker M, Alberti KGMM: Diabetic ketoacidosis and hyperglycaemic non-ketotic coma. In *International Textbook of Diabetes Mellitus.* Alberti KGMM, DeFronzo RA, Keen H, Zimmet P, Eds. Chichester, UK, Wiley, 1992, p. 1151–64

Rosenbloom AL: Intracerebral crises during treatment of diabetic ketoacidosis. *Diabetes Care* 13:22–33, 1990

Sperling MA: Diabetic ketoacidosis. *Pediatr Clin N Am* 31:591–610, 1984

Hypoglycemia

INTRODUCTION

The precise blood glucose level at which patients develop symptoms of hypoglycemia is difficult to define but, generally, symptoms do not occur until blood glucose is <50–60 mg/dl (<2.7–3.3 mM). Clinical hypoglycemia is the occurrence of typical autonomic and/or neuroglycopenic symptoms with low blood glucose levels, and its symptoms are relieved by the administration of carbohydrate. Because of its sporadic and somewhat unpredictable nature and because of the need for rapid treatment, hypoglycemia is often self-diagnosed on the basis of predominantly autonomic symptoms and may be treated without documentation of the blood glucose level.

PATHOPHYSIOLOGY

Hypoglycemia occurs when there is an imbalance between the rate of glucose removal from the circulation (e.g., uptake into muscle) and the rate of glucose entry into the circulation (e.g., release of glucose from the liver, or ingestion of nutrients). Clinically, this most often occurs when there is either

- a relative excess of insulin (which inhibits hepatic glucose production and stimulates glucose utilization by muscle and adipose tissue),
- a decrease or delay in food intake (which decreases the availability of dietary carbohydrate or gluconeogenic precursors), and/or
- an increase in the level of exercise (which accelerates glucose utilization by muscle).

In healthy individuals, as the glucose level declines below normal (typically to 50–60 mg/dl [2.7–3.3 mM]), a complex series of neuroendocrine events occur, which raise the plasma glucose concentration back toward normal. Glucagon and epinephrine are thought to be the most important counterregulatory hormones in this process because of their prompt secretion and potent ability to stimulate the release of glucose from the liver. In addition, epinephrine can contribute to glucose recovery by reducing glucose uptake into insulin-sensitive tissues, and it is responsible for many of the autonomic warning symptoms of hypoglycemia (see below). The other major counterregulatory hormones—cortisol and growth hormone—generally are released more slowly than glucagon and epinephrine and appear to have a more permissive role in glucose recovery. Finally, endogenous insulin secretion is typically inhibited by hypoglycemia, also facilitating the rise in plasma glucose levels.

In contrast, the patient with type I diabetes has several abnormalities in this feedback system. First, the secretion of glucagon typically becomes deficient within the first 2–5 yr of diabetes. Second, with more prolonged duration of disease, epinephrine secretion may also be impaired as a result of the development of subclinical autonomic neuropathy. Finally, the rate of absorption of insulin from a subcutaneous depot is not regulated by normal homeostatic mechanisms such as nutrient availability, and thus, it continues despite the presence of ongoing hypoglycemia. The combination of these and other factors makes the patient with type I diabetes particularly susceptible to the frequent development of hypoglycemia.

HYPOGLYCEMIA: MILD, MODERATE, AND SEVERE

Symptoms of Mild Reactions

Mild low blood glucose reactions usually consist of tremors, palpitations, sweating, and excessive hunger. These symptoms are mostly mediated through the autonomic (adrenergic) nervous system. Cognitive deficits usually do not accompany mild reactions, and patients are capable of self-treatment. These mild symptoms respond within 10–15 min after oral ingestion of 10–15 g of simple carbohydrate.

Symptoms of Moderate Reactions

Moderate low blood glucose reactions include neuroglycopenic as well as autonomic symptoms, e.g., headache, mood changes, irritability, decreased attentiveness, and drowsiness. Because of confusion, impaired judgment, and/or weakness, patients may require assistance in treating themselves. Moderate reactions produce longer-lasting and somewhat more severe symptoms and often require a second dose of simple carbohydrate.

Symptoms of Severe Reactions

Severe low blood glucose reactions are characterized by unresponsiveness, unconsciousness, or convulsions, and typically require assistance from another individual for appropriate treatment. Approximately 10% of type I diabetic patients suffer one severe reaction each year that requires emergency measures such as parenteral glucagon or intravenous glucose.

Potential Effects of Hypoglycemia

Mild hypoglycemic reactions may produce only minimal disruption of daily activities. Hypoglycemia can cause hunger with consequent overeating, thus contributing to obesity or hyperglycemia.

In contrast, moderate and severe reactions may be seriously disabling in many ways, and blood glucose levels should be kept high enough to avoid them. Hypoglycemia that interferes with normal thinking makes taking a school examination an impossible task; riding a bicycle, driving a car, or operating dangerous machinery become potentially disastrous. Repeated or prolonged episodes may cause irreparable damage to the CNS, especially in very young children. Finally, such reactions should be avoided because of their deleterious effects on the morale of the patient and family members.

Some patients develop either a fear of hypoglycemia or an inappropriate lack of concern. Fear of hypoglycemia can lead to chronic overeating, undertreatment with insulin, or both. Maintaining blood glucose levels of 240–400 mg/dl (13.3–22.2 mM) to avoid hypoglycemia increases the risk of metabolic complications, including diabetic ketoacidosis. In contrast, patients with a nonchalant attitude toward hypoglycemic reactions may maintain levels of blood glucose that are too low and will consequently be at greater risk for recurrent severe hypoglycemia. These patients can sometimes be identified by their near-normal glycohemoglobin levels.

Antecedents of Severe Hypoglycemia

Certain circumstances favor development of prolonged, incapacitating, and occasionally life-threatening hypoglycemia. Patients with hypoglycemia unawareness are always at increased risk for severe reactions. The counterregulatory hormone response to hypoglycemia and the autonomic symptoms tend to decrease after several years of diabetes so that neuroglycopenic symptoms become the first manifestation for many patients. β-Blockers and certain other medications may also diminish early warning signs.

Intensive insulin therapy also increases the risk of asymptomatic hypoglycemia. Although the increased frequency of low glucose levels can be attributed partly to the more stringent treatment goals associated with intensive regimens, it is now apparent that physiologic alterations occur in the patient's ability to secrete counterregulatory hormones, and thus, the ability to recognize and recover from hypoglycemia is clearly impaired. These observations emphasize the importance of SMBG in such patients to detect and prevent these asymptomatic reactions.

Several anecdotal and retrospective reports have suggested that the use of human insulin is associated with an increase in the frequency and severity of asymptomatic hypoglycemia. However, more carefully controlled, prospective studies generally have failed to support this observation. If a patient is switched from animal to human insulin, the health-care team should be aware that the more rapid onset of action and dissipation of human insulin may require readjustment of the insulin regimen or timing of meals to prevent hypoglycemia.

Delaying treatment is another common reason that mild hypoglycemia becomes more severe. Because early autonomic warning signs like headache, hunger, mood or behavior changes, or weakness are not specific to hypoglycemia, they are frequently misinterpreted or overlooked. This is especially likely if the patient's attention is directed elsewhere, which may occur during strenuous activity. Hypoglycemia during sleep is particularly difficult to detect. The patient should be questioned for the presence of nightmares or nocturnal diaphoresis, and family members should be alert to unusual sounds or activity during the patient's sleep.

COMMON CAUSES
OF HYPOGLYCEMIA

The factors precipitating an episode of hypoglycemia can often be identified by looking back over the events of several hours preceding the reactions (Table 4.7).

Inadvertent or deliberate errors in insulin dose are a frequent cause of hypoglycemia; other causes are changes in timing or schedule of insulin administration or meals. For example, sleeping later than usual is potentially dangerous for patients taking insulin because it disrupts the balance and timing between insulin and food. Changing insulin type to a more highly purified (and possibly more potent) preparation or from a mixed-species insulin to a purified pork or human insulin can cause hypoglycemia because of more rapid absorption or other factors (see above).

Vigorous unexpected exercise or activity is commonly associated with hypoglycemia. Aerobic exercise of prolonged duration or increased intensity can cause a reaction that occurs several hours after the activity period ends or even the next day.

Alcohol, marijuana, or other drugs often mask a patient's awareness of hypoglycemia in its earliest stages. By inhibiting the liver's gluconeogenic capacity, alcohol also prevents the body's normal ability to provide glucose and restore low glucose levels toward normal. Some of the most severe hypoglycemic reactions occur during or after parties because of the combination of physical activity and the use of alcohol or drugs can mask recognition of the problem and prevent the usual self-correction of hypoglycemia.

Anticipating and Preventing Hypoglycemia

Once a situation that leads to hypoglycemia is identified, adjustments can often be made to prevent future episodes.

Sleeping late. Although most patients can safely sleep an extra 30–45 min without particular adjustments, patients who oversleep >45 min need to plan in advance to alter insulin or food intake. For example, if sleeping late is anticipated, a 10–15% reduction of intermediate- or long-acting insulin on the previous evening is an effective means of preventing hypoglycemia. However, it may also lead to excessive morning hyperglycemia. When the patient awakens, the entire day's schedule of insulin and meals is advanced in time. Even the next day's schedule may be affected. All patients should be cautioned against awakening and taking insulin without eating and then resuming sleep. However, awakening early, performing a blood glucose test, administering insulin, eating breakfast, and then going back to sleep is generally safe. Patients treated with intensive therapy to achieve near-normal blood glucose levels may need to make adjustments in their basal and premeal bolus doses of insulin.

Exercise. To compensate for increased caloric needs of exercise, increased absorption of insulin from exercising muscles, and increased insulin sensitivity induced by extra activity, several strategies to prevent hypoglycemia can be employed. Most important, the exercising patient should always have a source of short-acting carbohydrate immediately available.

Table 4.7. Common Causes of Hypoglycemia

Insulin errors (inadvertent or deliberate)
- Reversal of morning and evening dosage
- Reversal of short- and intermediate-acting insulin
- Improper timing of insulin in relation to food
- Excessive insulin dosage

Intensive insulin therapy

Erratic or altered absorption of insulin
- More rapid absorption from exercising limbs
- Unpredictable absorption from hypertrophied injection sites

Use of more purified insulin preparations or changed from mixed species to singlespecies or human insulin

Nutrition
- Omitted or inadequate amounts of food
- Timing errors: late snacks or meals

Exercise
- Unplanned activity
- Prolonged duration or increased intensity of activity

Alcohol and drugs
- Impaired hepatic gluconeogenesis associated with alcohol intake
- Impaired mentation associated with alcohol, marijuana, or other illicit drugs

Role of SMBG

The availability of SMBG has made the detection and treatment of hypoglycemia practical, even in the subclinical range. Therefore, SMBG should be taught to all patients who do not already use it, and its frequency should be increased in patients with frequent hypoglycemia. Changes in insulin injection, eating or exercise schedules, travel, and other activities recognized as contributors to hypoglycemia call for increased frequency of monitoring. Patients should be instructed to treat asymptomatic hypoglycemia detected by SMBG.

TREATMENT

Mild Hypoglycemic Reactions

For mild reactions, 10–15 g of simple oral carbohydrate work quickly to increase the blood glucose and stop classic symptoms. Several sources of short-acting carbohydrate that will terminate mild hypoglycemic reactions include:
- 4–6 oz carbohydrate-containing liquids (e.g., unsweetened fruit juices, carbonated drinks),
- 5–6 LifeSavers candies,
- 1 tbsp of honey or Karo syrup,
- 4 tsp or packets of granulated sugar, or
- 6 1/2-inch sugar cubes.

Hypoglycemic reactions that occur during the night should be treated initially with 10–15 g of carbohydrate followed by a longer-acting mixture of carbohydrate and protein, e.g., 8 oz milk or 4 oz milk and a few crackers. This is intended to prevent further hypoglycemia during the night.

Commercially available glucose tablets have the added benefit of being premeasured to help prevent overtreatment. Glucose gels or small tubes of cake frosting are convenient for children or patients who are uncooperative when hypoglycemic. Chocolate and ice cream should be avoided for treating acute hypoglycemia because the fat content retards absorption of available sugar and could contribute to overweight from ingestion of unnecessary calories.

If early signs of hypoglycemia develop during exercise, the exercise should be halted and an appropriate amount of carbohydrate eaten (Table 2.5, page 27). If similar exercise has previously resulted in hypoglycemia, patients can anticipate and prevent it by snacking before, during, or after exercise, depending on when the episode occurred. Decisions regarding the type and time of extra food can be made based on SMBG (Table 3.6, page 49).

Alternatively, hypoglycemia can be prevented by anticipatory adjustments of insulin. For example, if a patient usually takes short-acting (regular) insulin before breakfast but is planning to exercise after breakfast, the insulin dose can be reduced by 10–20%. This strategy may be preferable for patients who do not want to increase the size of a meal before exercise or who are overweight.

Because there is always a risk that mild hypoglycemia will progress to a more severe reaction, all episodes must be treated promptly. Patients should be instructed never to continue driving when they begin to experience hypoglycemia. They should stop, treat the hypoglycemia, and wait 10–15 min to do a blood test to assure full recovery before they resume driving.

Moderate Hypoglycemia

Individuals with moderate reactions will often respond to the oral carbohydrates listed previously but may require more than one treatment and take longer to fully recover. These patients may be alert but will frequently be uncooperative or belligerent. Under such circumstances, if it becomes difficult to cajole the patient to take an oral carbohydrate, administration of subcutaneous or intramuscular glucagon may be more appropriate.

Severe Hypoglycemia

Patients with impaired consciousness or an inability to swallow may aspirate and should rarely be treated with oral carbohydrate. These patients require either parenteral glucagon or intravenous glucose. If these are not available, glucose gels, applied between the patient's cheek and gum, may be of some help.

Generally, clinical improvement should occur within 10–15 min after glucagon injection and within 1–5 min of intravenous glucose administration. However, if hypoglycemia was prolonged or extremely severe, complete recovery of normal mental function may not occur for hours. Repeated boluses of intravenous glucose do not hasten recovery unless blood glucose measurements show persistent hypoglycemia. If the hypoglycemic event was associated with convulsions, the postictal period may be associated with severe headaches, lethargy, amnesia, or vomiting. Decreased muscle control may also be seen and requires medical evaluation if it persists.

Recurrent episodes of severe hypoglycemia can lead to permanent cognitive deficits. To prevent recurrence, patients should eat their planned meal or snack (~10% of daily calories) after initial treatment of moderate or severe reactions or when treating any nocturnal reaction.

Glucagon. The dose of glucagon needed to treat moderate or severe hypoglycemia for a child <5 yr old is 0.25–0.50 mg; for an older child (5–10 yr), 0.50–1 mg; and for those >10 yr old, 1 mg. Glucagon should be given intramuscularly or subcutaneously in the deltoid or anterior thigh region. Parents, roommates, and spouses should be taught how to mix, draw up, and administer glucagon so that they are properly prepared for emergency situations. Kits that include a syringe prefilled with diluting fluid are available.

Intravenous glucose. If medical staff and equipment are available, intravenous glucose should be given as a primary treatment in preference to glucagon. The usual dose is 10–25 g administered as 50% dextrose over 1–3 min. The dose can be titrated according to the patient's response. After the bolus injection, intravenous glucose (5–10 g/h) should be continued until the patient has fully recovered and is able to eat.

HYPOGLYCEMIA UNAWARENESS

In the Diabetes Control and Complications Trial (DCCT), about one third of all episodes of severe hypoglycemia seen in awake, intensively treated patients were not accompanied by sufficient signs or symptoms so that patients could effectively prevent neuroglycopenia. In the past, hypoglycemia without warning was viewed as a rare condition associated with advanced autonomic neuropathy. This concept is incorrect. Forms of hypoglycemia without warning can occur in recently diagnosed patients, particularly in patients with repeated episodes of recent hypoglycemia and low HbA_{1c} concentrations. Repeated episodes of hypoglycemia cause two problems. First, they blunt hormonal defense mechanisms that prevent hypoglycemia. Second, they lower the level at which early hypoglycemic symptoms are perceived.

The key clinical issue is that patients need to be reminded that the absence of symptoms of hypoglycemia when glucose level is <55 mg/dl (<3.1 mM) should prompt consultation with an experienced physician. Increased reliance on more frequent blood glucose monitoring, particularly before driving and after strenuous exercise, should be considered. Recent evidence suggests that hypoglycemia unawareness can be reversed by intensive education and self-management training and efforts that successfully avoid hypoglycemia. These efforts may include adapting slightly higher blood glucose targets before meals and during the night and self-management training to help detect and prevent subtle early signs of hypoglycemia.

HYPOGLYCEMIA WITH SUBSEQUENT HYPERGLYCEMIA

Hypoglycemia followed by "rebound" hyperglycemia, also called the Somogyi effect, may complicate diabetes management in some patients. The phenomenon originates during hypoglycemia, with the secretion of counterregulatory hormones (glucagon, epinephrine, growth hormone, and cortisol). This hormonal surge, together with decreasing insulin levels, leaves counterregulatory hormones relatively unopposed. Hepatic glucose production is stimulated, thereby raising blood glucose levels. These hormones may cause some insulin resistance for a 12- to 48-h period. Moreover, excessive carbohydrate intake may be a major contributor to rebound hyperglycemia.

The frequency of this phenomenon is debated, and recent studies suggest that it is much less common than previously reported. It may follow nocturnal hypoglycemia, but it also may occur after hypoglycemia at any time. The hypoglycemic event that precedes the rebound may not produce sufficient symptoms to make it recognizable.

If rebound hyperglycemia goes unrecognized and insulin dosage is increased, a cycle of overinsulinization may result, i.e., more hypoglycemia, more rebound hyperglycemia, more insulin, more hypoglycemia. As a general rule, when hyperglycemia does not respond as expected to treatment adjustments, undetected hypoglycemia and rebound hyperglycemia should be considered as a possible explanation. Rather than increasing insulin dosage day after day, the clinician who suspects rebound hyperglycemia should endeavor to detect (via SMBG) and avoid the initiating hypoglycemic event.

Nocturnal rebound hyperglycemia should be investigated by measuring blood glucose levels between 0200 and 0400 and again at 0700. If blood glucose levels between 0200 and 0400 are <50–60 mg/dl (<2.8–3.3 mM) and those at 0700 are >180–200 mg/dl (>10.0–11.1 mM), rebound hyperglycemia may have occurred. The increased blood glucose level may be exacerbated by the waning effect of the previous dose of intermediate-acting insulin or a prominent dawn phenomenon (see below). A decrease in presupper intermediate-acting insulin or its deferral to ~2100 or an appropriate change in bedtime snack should prevent nocturnal hypoglycemia.

DAWN AND PREDAWN PHENOMENA

The amount of insulin required to normalize blood glucose during the night is less in the predawn period (0100–0300) than at dawn (0500–0800). The modest (20–40 mg/dl [1.1–2.2 mM]) increase in plasma glucose commonly seen in patients with type I diabetes given enough insulin to avoid hypoglycemia in the predawn period is referred to as the dawn phenomenon. This increment can be greater if insulin levels decline between the predawn and dawn periods or if hypoglycemia occurs during the predawn period. The key clinical implication is that attempts to normalize prebreakfast glucose level (i.e., 70–115 mg/dl [3.9–6.4 mM]) often result in early-morning hypoglycemia.

Several strategies can be used to identify and prevent nocturnal hypoglycemia. These should include monitoring blood glucose at bedtime and at 0200–0300, especially when insulin doses are being adjusted to correct prebreakfast hyperglycemia or when blood glucose level is frequently in the normoglycemic range before breakfast. In the DCCT, >50% of all episodes of severe hypoglycemia occurred during the night or when patients were asleep, even with the use of long-acting insulin preparations given at night or insulin infusion pumps. As a consequence, the medium blood glucose before breakfast was 140 mg/dl (7.8 mM), and >75% of all pre-breakfast values were over the upper target range of 120 mg/dl (6.7 mM). Adding extra food at bedtime (particularly protein, which helps stimulate glucagon secretion) and giving insulin that does not "peak" at 0100–0300 should be considered. Increasing the bedtime snack is particularly important when nocturnal hypoglycemia is most likely (e.g., after sustained exercise during the day or when prebedtime glucose is <100 mg/dl (<5.6 mM). Among patients taking twice-daily injections, giving the evening intermediate-acting insulin at bedtime or substituting it with long-acting insulin may be effective. Patients using infusion pumps can also preprogram these to give less insulin during the predawn hours and more at dawn.

CONCLUSION

Severe hypoglycemia can be life threatening if not treated promptly. Even mild and moderate hypoglycemia can cause both short- and long-term problems. All patients should be taught to be aware of the signs of hypoglycemia and should be encouraged to use SMBG more frequently to prevent and monitor episodes. All families should be taught how to use glucagon and when to call for medical assistance.

BIBLIOGRAPHY

Amiel SA, Tamborlane WV, Sacca L, Sherwin RS: Hypoglycemia and glucose counterregulation in normal and insulin-dependent diabetic subjects. *Diabetes Metab Rev* 4:71–89, 1988

Bolli GB, Perriello G, Fanelli CG, De Feo P: Nocturnal blood glucose control in type I diabetes mellitus. *Diabetes Care* 16 (Suppl. 3): 71–89, 1993

Clarke WL, Gonder-Frederick LA, Richards FE, Cryer PE: Multifactorial origin of hypoglycemic symptom unawareness in IDDM: association with defective glucose counterregulation and better glycemic control. *Diabetes* 40: 680–85, 1991

Cryer PE: Hypoglycemia unawareness in IDDM. *Diabetes Care* 16 (Suppl. 3): 40–47, 1993

Cryer PE, Fisher JN, Shamoon H: Hypoglycemia (technical review). *Diabetes Care*. In press

Cryer PE, Gerich JE: Glucose counterregulation, hypoglycemia and intensive insulin therapy in diabetes mellitus. *N Engl J Med* 313:232–41, 1985

DCCT Research Group: Epidemiology of severe hypoglycemia in the diabetes control and complications trial. *Am J Med* 90:450–59, 1991

Fanelli CG, Epifano L, Rambotti AM, Pampanelli S, Di Vincenzo A, Modarelli F, Lepore M, Annibale B, Ciofetta M, Bottini P, Porcellati F, Scionti L, Santeusanio F, Brunetti P, Bolli GB: Meticulous prevention of hypoglycemia normalizes the glycemic thresholds and magnitude of most of neuroendocrine responses to, symptoms of, and cognitive function during hypoglycemia in intensively treated patients with short-term IDDM. *Diabetes* 42: 1683–89, 1993

Havlin CE, Cryer PE: Nocturnal hypoglycemia does not commonly result in major morning hyperglycemia in patients with diabetes mellitus. *Diabetes Care* 2:141–47, 1987

Widom B, Simonson DC: Glycemic control and neuropsychologic function during hypoglycemia in patients with insulin-dependent diabetes mellitus. *Ann Intern Med* 112:904–12, 1990

Pregnancy

INTRODUCTION

Type I diabetes mellitus complicates ~0.1–0.5% of all pregnancies. During the past 15 yr, perinatal outcome has improved remarkably in this high-risk group. Except for deaths due to major fetal malformations, the perinatal mortality rate for women with diabetes who receive optimal care now approaches that of the general obstetric population.

Management of the patient with type I diabetes during pregnancy ideally involves an experienced health-care team, including the internist or endocrinologist, obstetrician or maternal-fetal specialist, pediatrician or neonatologist, teaching nurse, dietitian, the patient, and her partner. Experience indicates that the outcome for both mother and baby is generally more favorable when an experienced team is responsible for management during pregnancy, delivery, and the perinatal period. When a team is not conveniently available, phone consultation with individual specialists is helpful.

Pregnant women are usually highly motivated; therefore, this time is ideal for teaching self-care skills they can use for the rest of their lives.

RISK FACTORS

What factors help quantify maternal and fetal risk in the diabetic pregnancy? Generally, risk factors fall into two categories: those relating to diabetes and its control and those relating to vascular complications. Thus, pregnancies complicated by type I diabetes can be divided into two groups: women with diabetes, and women with diabetes and vascular complications.

Diabetes and Its Control

The earlier the onset of diabetes and the longer its duration, the worse the prognosis for good perinatal outcome. The quality of maternal glucose control throughout pregnancy is also an important consideration. Ketoacidosis and associated intrauterine deaths are most common in patients with poor blood glucose control.

Vasculopathy

The greater the degree of vasculopathy, the greater the likelihood of a poor outcome for mother and child. Nephropathy, particularly if associated with hypertension, appears to bring the greatest hazards, increasing the risk of preeclampsia, fetal-growth retardation, and preterm delivery. Pregnancy can contribute to a worsening of retinal disease in women with background or proliferative retinopathy, especially in the presence of hypertension; women with active proliferative retinopathy are at greatest risk for loss of visual acuity. Maternal deaths have been reported in patients with coronary artery disease. Other prognostically bad signs during pregnancy include ketoacidosis, pyelonephritis, preeclampsia, and poor clinic attendance or neglect.

MATERNAL METABOLISM DURING PREGNANCY

During gestation, maternal metabolism adapts to provide the fetus with an uninterrupted supply of fuel. During the first and second trimesters of a normal pregnancy, accelerated utilization of glucose by the developing fetus generally produces a decrease in maternal glucose levels. In women with type I diabetes, insulin requirements may decrease. Later in gestation, insulin resistance produced by the changing hormonal milieu may increase glucose levels in nondiabetic women. In women with diabetes, this may result in an increased insulin requirement.

In nondiabetic women, estrogen and progesterone alter maternal islet cell function, producing β-cell hyperplasia and contributing to maternal hyperinsulinemia. In addition, maternal cortisol is elevated during pregnancy, which potentiates glucose intolerance. Human placental lactogen (hPL), a growth hormone-like protein synthesized by the placental syncytiotrophoblast, produces insulin resistance and augments maternal lipolysis. As placental mass enlarges during pregnancy, hPL levels rise, allowing increased maternal utilization of fats for energy and sparing of glucose for fetal consumption. In late pregnancy, the progression of overnight maternal fasting ketosis is so accelerated that delaying breakfast may result in significant ketonuria.

In pregnancy complicated by diabetes, periods of maternal hyperglycemia produce fetal hyperglycemia. Larger amounts of maternal amino acids and other fuels also cross to the fetus. Elevated levels of maternal glucose and other nutrients stimulate the fetal pancreas, resulting in β-cell hyperplasia and hyperinsulinemia. This combination of fetal overnutrition and fetal hyperinsulinemia contributes to morbidity and mortality observed in the infant of the diabetic mother.

CARE BEFORE CONCEPTION

Treatment of the patient with type I diabetes must begin before gestation (Table 4.8). For this reason, any regular visit to the physician by a reproductive-age woman, from teenage to middle age, should be considered a preconception visit. These contacts provide an important opportunity to discuss the patient's contraceptive needs and her thoughts and concerns about a future pregnancy and to establish a data base that can be used in assessing perinatal risk. Adolescents in particular should be encouraged to discuss these issues routinely with members of the health-care team.

Important periodic assessments include measurements of blood pressure, an ophthalmologic examination, an electrocardiogram, and a 24-h urine collection for creatinine clearance and protein excretion. Glycated hemoglobin should be performed routinely, and self-monitoring of blood glucose (SMBG) taught, if needed.

Immune status against rubella should also be checked before conception. Consultation with a nutritionist and a review of the patient's exercise program are important. The patient must understand

that smoking and alcohol are strictly prohibited during pregnancy.

Because pregnancy complicated by type I diabetes may cause emotional and financial stress, it is essential to evaluate the psychosocial interactions of the patient and her partner, their support network, and their financial resources.

PRECONCEPTION COUNSELING

Women with type I diabetes who are contemplating pregnancy often have questions regarding its impact on their health and the possible consequences for the fetus. Some of the most commonly encountered questions, along with suggested answers, are presented below:

Q. How will pregnancy affect my life expectancy?

A. Pregnancy is not generally life threatening, but serious complications can occur. There is no evidence that pregnancy shortens the lives of women with type I diabetes, except for those with established coronary artery disease. However, women with diabetes do face a higher risk for certain complications. If ketoacidosis occurs, it is

---

TABLE 4.8. Care Before Conception

■ Discuss contraceptive program
■ Establish data base for perinatal risk
  ■ Assess vascular status:
    Ophthalmologic examination
    ECG
    24-h urine for protein
    Creatinine clearance
    Check all peripheral pulses
  ■ Assess glycemic control via glycated hemoglobin
■ Optimize glycemic control; teach SMBG if needed
■ Refer for assessment of nutritional adequacy; adjust if needed
■ Determine immune status against rubella
■ Evaluate psychosocial setting
  ■ Caution patient against smoking or excessive alcohol
  ■ Assess exercise program

SMBG, self-monitoring of blood glucose.

likely to be more dangerous during pregnancy; and both preeclampsia and delivery by cesarean section are more common in diabetic women.

Q. What effect will pregnancy have on diabetic nephropathy?

A. There is no evidence that pregnancy will permanently worsen diabetic nephropathy, although a temporary increase in proteinuria and decrease in creatinine clearance may occur. On the other hand, advanced nephropathy may jeopardize both mother and infant. Severe diabetic nephropathy may increase the likelihood of early delivery and/or a smaller-than-normal infant. Factors that point in this direction include
■ proteinuria >3 g/24 h in the 1st trimester or >10 g/24 h in the 3rd trimester,
■ serum creatinine >1.5 mg/dl at the start of pregnancy,
■ hematocrit <25% in the 3rd trimester, and
■ hypertension.

Q. What effect will pregnancy have on diabetic retinopathy?

A. Except for women with active proliferative retinopathy, pregnancy is usually an ophthalmologically stable period. Women without diabetic retinopathy will not usually develop it during pregnancy. Very few women who have background retinopathy at the start of pregnancy experience a worsening of this condition and very rarely to a proliferative stage. Proliferative retinopathy treated by laser photocoagulation and stable before pregnancy will generally remain so. In contrast, many women with active proliferative retinopathy that has not been treated with photocoagulation experience a serious worsening of this complication during pregnancy.

Q. Will the baby develop diabetes mellitus?

A. Although the infant is slightly more likely to develop type I diabetes, the risk is not very high—~1% if the mother is ≥25 yr old at child's birth and ~4% if the mother is <25 yr old at child's birth. These risks are doubled if the mother was diagnosed before age 11.

Q. Can I use birth control pills?

A. Young women without vascular complications may use a low-dose estrogen (≤35 μg)/progestin oral contraceptive. Those with hypertension or vasculopathy should use a progestin-only pill (or some other means of birth control).

Q. What effect will diabetes have on the baby?

A. The answer to this question appears to hinge largely on the mother's blood glucose control; generally, the better the diabetes control, the fewer the complications. In the first weeks of pregnancy, poor diabetes control appears to increase the occurrence of fetal malformations. Later, high blood glucose levels may bring about other serious consequences. Because glucose crosses from the mother to the fetus but insulin does not, high maternal glucose stimulates the fetus to overproduce insulin, which may
■ cause excessive fetal growth,
■ prevent the baby's lungs (and other organs) from maturing at a normal pace, or
■ give the baby serious hypoglycemia after birth, when it no longer receives glucose from the mother.
In addition, high glucose levels are associated with sudden unexplained fetal death late in pregnancy.

CONGENITAL MALFORMATIONS: RISK AND DETECTION

The incidence of major congenital malformations is typically increased in the offspring of patients with type I diabetes over the 2–3% rate observed in the general population. However, the rate may vary considerably—from <5% in patients with excellent glycemic control before conception to as high as 20–25% among women with markedly elevated glycated hemoglobin in the 1st trimester.

Steadily accumulating evidence links such malformations with inadequate diabetes control during embryogenesis (gestational wk 3–7). For this reason, patients should be as near euglycemia as possible at the time of conception and throughout the 1st trimester. All women of childbearing age should be made aware of these risks, and if pregnancy is considered, they should be encouraged to use contraception until excellent glycemic control is achieved (see PHILOSOPHY AND GOALS). The risk of fetal anomalies should be reviewed at the first prenatal visit.

Many fetal anomalies, particularly in the CNS, heart, skeleton, and urinary tract, may be detected before birth. The evaluation for a potential fetal malformation should include a maternal serum α-fetoprotein level at 16 wk, a detailed ultrasound examination of fetal anatomy at 16–18 wk, and an assessment of fetal cardiac structure by echocardiography at 20 wk (Table 4.9). All of these studies require interpretation by individuals experienced in prenatal diagnosis.

MATERNAL GLUCOSE CONTROL DURING PREGNANCY

It is generally accepted that excellent control of maternal diabetes will reduce the risks of fetal demise, excessive fetal growth, and delayed pulmonary maturation. During a nondiabetic pregnancy, maternal plasma glucose rarely exceeds 100 mg/dl (5.6 mM), ranging from fasting levels of 60 mg/dl (3.3 mM) to postprandial levels of 120 mg/dl (6.7 mM). These values should be therapeutic objectives for pregnancies complicated by type I diabetes (Table 4.10).

Maintaining maternal glucose levels in this range throughout gestation is difficult. During the 1st trimester, when morning sickness may be troublesome, the risk of hypoglycemia is increased; hypoglycemia is most likely during the night, when the mother is fasting but the fetus and placenta continue to consume glucose. In contrast, during the early 3rd trimester, when the diabetogenic stress of pregnancy is greatest, insulin needs may rise 50% over 4–6 wk, heightening the risk for ketoacidosis.

Monitoring Control

SMBG. During pregnancy, women with type I diabetes must use SMBG to assess control. SMBG has been shown to decrease the need for hospitalization and reduce the cost of care. Patients should monitor in the fasting state, before each meal, and possibly 1–2 h after meals. Testing at 0200–0300 is necessary for patients who are likely to experience nocturnal hypoglycemia, those who have persistent fasting hyperglycemia, or those who are using continuous subcutaneous insulin-infusion (CSII) pump treatment. The patient should be instructed to maintain a careful record of her daily glucose values with comments about calorie intake and exercise.

Available data are too limited to permit specific recommendations regarding exercise programs in pregnant women with diabetes. However, a regular program of moderate-intensity aerobic exercise does not appear to have adverse effects and may help improve maternal glucose control and sense of well-being.

Glycated hemoglobin. A glycated hemoglobin determination should be obtained at the patient's first prenatal

---

Table 4.9. Fetal Evaluation

Midpregnancy (16–20 wk): to detect fetal anomalies
- Maternal serum α-fetoprotein
- Ultrasonography
- Fetal echocardiography

Late pregnancy (28 wk to delivery): to assess fetal well-being
- Maternal assessment of fetal activity
- Nonstress test
- Contraction stress test
- Fetal biophysical profile
- Ultrasonography
- Lecithin-to-sphingomyelin (L/S) ratio, lung profile

Table 4.10. Target Blood Glucose Levels in Pregnancy

TIME OF MEASUREMENT	BLOOD GLUCOSE
Before breakfast	60–90 mg/dl (3.3–5 mM)
Before lunch, supper, and bedtime snack	60–105 mg/dl (3.3–5.8 mM)
2 h after meals	≤120 mg/dl (≤6.7 mM)
0200–0600	≥60 mg/dl (≥3.3 mM)

Glycated hemoglobin levels should be within the normal range for the individual laboratory.

visit to assess previous glycemic control. This test should be repeated every 4–6 wk.

Urine testing. Although the increased glomerular filtration rate of pregnancy limits the value of urinary glucose testing, patients should be instructed to test urine for ketones before breakfast every day and if capillary glucose levels at any time exceed 200 mg/dl (>11.1 mM).

Insulin Regimen During Pregnancy

An insulin regimen tailored to the patient's needs can be developed based on SMBG data, the meal plan, and the exercise regimen. Most women will require at least two daily injections of a mixture of intermediate-acting (NPH, lente) and short-acting (regular) insulins. Patients usually received two-thirds of the total insulin dose at breakfast and the remaining third at supper. The morning combination ordinarily contains twice as much intermediate-acting as short-acting insulin, and the evening dose is divided equally between the two.

Delaying the evening intermediate-acting component until near bedtime may help to avoid glycemic irregularities overnight. In this case, the morning injection remains the same, but short-acting insulin alone is given at supper and intermediate-acting insulin alone at bedtime. Postponing the intermediate-acting component decreases the likelihood of nocturnal hypoglycemia and may provide effective prophylactic treat-

ment for the dawn phenomenon and/or the waning of the insulin effect in the early morning hours leading to pre-breakfast hyperglycemia (see HYPO-GLYCEMIA, pages 88–89).

Some patients prefer the flexibility of a four-injection regimen: short-acting insulin at breakfast, lunch, and supper, with an injection of intermediate- or long-acting (ultralente) insulin at bedtime.

In general, if glucose levels remains elevated, the corresponding insulin dose is increased by 20%.

Continuous subcutaneous insulin infusion. Selected patients who have used pump therapy before gestation may be continued on this program. However, this treatment appears to offer no significant advantage over multiple insulin injections and may actually increase risk of ketoacidosis secondary to pump malfunction. The nocturnal basal infusion dose must often be decreased to reduce the risk of hypoglycemia, and ketoacidosis and intrauterine fetal death can occur in association with pump failure or maternal infection.

NUTRITION NEEDS

The daily nutrition needs of pregnant women with type I diabetes should be based on a nutrition assessment by a dietitian. SMBG results, urine ketones, appetite, and weight gain can be a guide to developing and evaluating an individualized meal plan.

For most patients, 10% of the calories should be consumed at breakfast, 30% at lunch, and 30% at supper. The remaining 30% of calories can be distributed among several snacks, particularly a bedtime snack to decrease the risk of nocturnal hypoglycemia. Additional snacks may be added if the patients anticipates an increase in exercise. Patients with persistently elevated mid-morning glucose levels should reduce the calorie content of breakfast and redistribute the calories to lunch and supper. The presence of morning ketonuria with normal glucose levels indicates the need to increase the calorie content of the bedtime snack or to consider adding an 0300 snack. The calorie content of the meal plan may be reduced in women who are obese, who demonstrate early excessive weight gain, or who have a sedentary lifestyle. Guidelines for calorie needs for women who begin pregnancy at desirable weight can be obtained from appropriate references (see also NUTRITION, page 62).

OUTPATIENT CARE

Most women with type I diabetes may be managed as outpatients throughout gestation. Some may benefit from early hospitalization to evaluate cardiovascular and renal status and glucose control. In addition, failure to maintain acceptable glucose levels, worsening hypertension, or infectious complications such as a viral illness or pyelonephritis may necessitate hospitalization. A urine culture should be ordered in the 1st trimester.

Clinic visits can be scheduled at 1- to 2-wk intervals for most women. At each visit, the patient's SMBG log should be reviewed, problems with hyperglycemia and/or hypoglycemia discussed, and the patient's weight gain and blood pressure checked. The patient should also be instructed to telephone the physician promptly if there are any episodes of hypoglycemia (<50 mg/dl [<2.8 mM]) or hyperglycemia (>200 mg/dl [>11.1 mM]) so that appropriate remedial action may be taken.

Throughout gestation, the physician coordinating the patient's management must communicate regularly with other members of the health-care team. If background retinopathy has been detected, repeat ophthalmologic examinations should be obtained in the 2nd or 3rd trimester; proliferative retinopathy requires more intensive follow-up. Renal function studies including creatinine clearance and protein excretion should be repeated in each trimester.

Assessment of Fetal Condition

Significant advances have been made in the ability to assess fetal growth and well-being. The detection of fetal malformations between 16 and 20 wk is discussed on page 93. In the 3rd trimester, attention should be directed toward the assessment of fetal well-being, growth, and pulmonary maturation (Table 4.9). Several approaches should be used to assess fetal condition to prevent sudden intrauterine death, a catastrophe most likely to occur during the final 4–6 wk of gestation.

Patient self-assessment. Maternal monitoring of fetal activity has proved to be a simple yet valuable screening approach in high-risk pregnancies. Daily assessment of fetal movement may be started at 28 wk gestation. The patient counts fetal activity for several 30- to 60-min periods throughout the day or records the time of day at which she has felt a total of 10 fetal movements. A significant decrease in fetal activity demands further evaluation.

Nonstress test. The nonstress test (NST) is an ideal screening technique that is easily performed in an outpatient setting and usually requires no more than 20 min. Fetal heart rate is recorded with an external heart rate monitor. A normal response is the presence of two or more accelerations of at least 15 beats and lasting at least 15 s during 20 min of observation. This "reactive" test is considered a reassuring finding. In a metabolically stable patient, a reactive NST will predict fetal survival for up to 1 wk.

The NST may be performed weekly after 28 wk of gestation and then twice weekly at 32 wk of gestation. Because normal fetal activity and a reactive NST are rarely associated with an intrauterine fetal death, the primary value of surveillance is to allow the clinician to delay delivery safely while the fetus gains further maturity. However, because the screening tests have significant false-positive rates, an abnormal test, e.g., as a decrease in fetal activity, must be further evaluated.

Contraction stress test. The contraction stress test, in which uterine contractions are induced and the response of the fetal heart rate to the contractions is observed, may be required if the NST is nonreactive or suggests fetal compromise.

Biophysical profile. Some clinicians have turned to the biophysical profile to assess fetal condition. The biophysical profile utilizes real-time ultrasound to observe fetal activity, fetal breathing movements, amniotic fluid volume, and fetal tone. Like the NST, the biophysical profile can usually be completed in 15 min and, if normal, indicates fetal well-being.

Assessment of Fetal Growth

Fetal growth should be assessed with serial ultrasound examinations every 4–6 wk. Delivery by cesarian section should be considered if the ultrasound suggests excessive fetal size.

The techniques utilized today for antepartum fetal surveillance permit most patients to remain outside the hospital even during the final 4–6 wk of gestation, as long as maternal control is acceptable and fetal evaluation is reassuring. Nevertheless, hospitalization may be necessary if the patient has nephropathy and/or hypertension, if she has not adhered to the regimen, or when fetal jeopardy is suspected.

TIMING OF DELIVERY

In the past, preterm delivery was often elected to avoid the risk of intrauterine fetal death. In many instances, such infants, although born alive, succumbed to respiratory distress syndrome (RDS). An increased incidence of RDS due to the combined effects of prematurity and diabetes, which may retard normal maturation of pulmonary surfactant production, was observed in infants of diabetic mothers.

Today, delivery can be safely delayed until term in most pregnancies complicated by type I diabetes. Labor may then be induced when the cervix is favorable, or the onset of spontaneous labor may be awaited. Patients must continue excellent glycemic control, and all parameters of antepartum fetal surveillance should remain normal.

In women who have vasculopathy, who have been in poor control, who have had a prior stillbirth, or who have not adhered to the program of care, early elective delivery to prevent a late fetal death may be planned provided that fetal pulmonary maturation has been confirmed by the analysis of amniotic fluid

for surfactant. RDS is highly unlikely when the amniotic fluid lecithin-to-sphingomyelin (L/S) ratio is ≥2.0 and the acidic phospholipid phosphatidylglycerol is present.

If the fetal lungs are still immature at 38 wk, delivery may be postponed as long as the results of fetal assessment remains reassuring. In such cases, amniocentesis may be repeated in ~1 wk. It is essential that the obstetrician know the reliability of the analytical technique used for phospholipid analysis in the reporting laboratory, particularly in pregnancies complicated by diabetes mellitus.

Delivery despite fetal lung immaturity may be necessary when testing suggests fetal compromise or if the pregnant patient develops preeclampsia, rapidly worsening retinopathy, or renal failure.

LABOR AND DELIVERY

The timing and site of delivery must be discussed and coordinated with the neonatologists who are to be present. If delivery is anticipated and adequate maternal or neonatal care cannot be provided, the patient should be transferred to a hospital with an appropriately equipped nursery. Expert care is required to deal with the various complications that may arise in the infant of the diabetic mother.

Intrapartum electronic monitoring of the fetal heart rate is mandatory. Labor should be allowed to progress as long as cervical dilation and descent follow the established curves for normal labor. Any evidence of an arrest pattern should alert the physician to the possibility of cephalopelvic disproportion and fetal macrosomia.

Maternal Glucose Levels During Delivery

Maintenance of normal maternal glucose levels (60–100 mg/dl [3.3–5.6 mM]) during labor and delivery will reduce the risk of subsequent neonatal hypoglycemia. During active labor in most patients, insulin requirements typically decrease substantially. Glucose levels should be determined hourly with SMBG techniques at the bedside, because even small doses of insulin may produce hypoglycemia during active labor. Adjustments in the delivery of insulin and/or glucose should be made based on the glucose determinations.

If labor is electively induced or a cesarean section is planned, the procedure should be schedule for the early morning, and the patient's usual morning insulin dose should be withheld. Epidural anesthesia is preferred in patients scheduled for cesarean section. After the operation has been completed, glucose levels should be monitored every 1–2 h, and an intravenous solution containing 5% dextrose should be continued. Because hPL and its contrainsulin actions fall rapidly after removal of the placenta, no insulin may be required for the remainder of the day.

POSTPARTUM CARE

In the immediate postpartum period, the patient's insulin requirements are usually lower than her prepregnancy needs. The antepartum objective of physiologic glycemic control is usually relaxed at this time. Breastfeeding is encouraged. The meal plan for the breastfeeding mother should be 33–37 kcal/kg desirable body weight.

If the patient delivered vaginally, and if glucose levels are $\geq$200 mg/dl ($\geq$11.1 mM), short-acting insulin may be administered as necessary on the first and second postpartum days. On days 3 and 4, insulin dosage is based on the total insulin needed on days 1 and 2; the patient should be given two-thirds of this total dose as intermediate-acting insulin, supplemented by short-acting insulin as determined by SMBG.

In patients who have undergone a cesarean section, little or no insulin may be required for the first 2 or 3 postoperative days because calorie intake is limited. On days 3 and 4, short-acting insulin may be administered for glucose levels $\geq$200 mg/dl ($\geq$11.1 mM), and the following day, two thirds of the daily total may be administered as intermedi-ate acting insulin supplemented by short-acting insulin as indicated by SMBG. Adjustment of insulin needs in the postpartum period should always be individualized based on SMBG results.

FAMILY PLANNING AND CONTRACEPTION

Family planning and contraception must be reviewed with the patient during the postpartum period. Although oral contraceptives are the most effective method available, the increased risk of thromboembolic disease and vasculopathy require that combined estrogen/progestin oral-contraceptive preparations be used with caution; only low-dose ($\leq$35 µg) estrogen agents should be prescribed. Combination agents are contraindicated in women with hypertension or vasculopathy, who may be offered a progestin-only pill instead.

Motivated patients may do well with one of the barrier methods of contraception, such as the diaphragm, although their efficacy is significantly lower than that of oral contraceptives. Sterilization should be discussed with the patient when she has completed her family or if she has serious vasculopathy.

CONCLUSION

Advances in biochemical and electronic monitoring techniques have markedly improved maternal and fetal well-being in pregnancy complicated by diabetes. Meticulous metabolic control before and during pregnancy holds the key to a successful outcome and to minimizing fetal malformations or neonatal complications. A team approach is more likely to achieve a desirable result.

BIBLIOGRAPHY

Daly A: Nutrition management. In *Therapy for Diabetes Mellitus and Related Disorders*. Lebovitz H, Ed. Alexandria, VA, Am. Diabetes Assoc., 1994

Freinkel N, Dooley SL, Metzger BE: Care of the pregnant woman with insulin-dependent diabetes mellitus. *N Engl J Med* 313:96–103, 1985

Gabbe SG: Management of diabetes mellitus in pregnancy. *Am J Obstet Gynecol* 153:824–28, 1985

Jovanovic L, Fuhrmann K, Peterson CM: *Diabetes in Pregnancy: Teratology, Toxicology, and Treatment.* New York, Praeger, 1985

Kitzmiller JL, Gavin LA, Gin GD, Jovanovic-Peterson L, Main EK, Zigrang WD: Preconception care of diabetes: glycemic control prevents congenital anomalies. *JAMA* 265:731–36, 1991

Medical Management of Pregnancy Complicated by Diabetes. Jovanovic-Peterson L, Ed. Alexandria, VA, Am. Diabetes Assoc., 1993

Rizzo T, Metzger BE, Burns WJ, Burns K: Correlations between antepartum maternal metabolism and intelligence of offspring. *N Engl J Med* 325: 911–16, 1991

Surgery

INTRODUCTION

The physician caring for patients with type I diabetes mellitus should become familiar with proper pre- and postoperative management during elective or emergency surgery. It is now possible for a patient with diabetes to undergo surgery with little more than normal risk, given sufficient time for complete patient evaluation and preparation. Guidelines for diabetes management during both elective and emergency surgery are presented herein.

GENERAL PRINCIPLES

The objectives of glycemic management before, during, and after an operation are to prevent hypoglycemia as well as excessive hyperglycemia and ketoacidosis. Insulin requirements often increase during the acute stress of a major surgical procedure, despite the fact that the patient may not be eating. For this reason, the patient's customary basal insulin dosage is usually continued throughout the perioperative period. Supplemental insulin also may be needed to prevent excessive hepatic glucose release and decreased peripheral utilization with resulting hyperglycemia. Normal fluid and electrolyte balance should be maintained, and oral feedings should be resumed as soon as possible.

Although, ideally, plasma glucose level should be maintained near that of nondiabetic individuals at all times, precision of control is difficult to achieve in practice and increases the risk of hypoglycemia; therefore, it is generally considered safer to err on the side of mild hyperglycemia. Although some evidence suggests that perioperative hyperglycemia may delay healing, the risks are small compared with those of hypoglycemia in a patient whose mental status is already altered by anesthesia or postoperative medications.

Plasma glucose levels between 150 and 250 mg/dl (8.3–13.9 mM) during and after the operation are considered satisfactory. With a highly skilled operative/postoperative team and readily available monitoring, blood glucose levels may be targeted to remain between 120 and 180 mg/dl (6.7 and 10.0 mM).

Medical management of the patient with diabetes will depend on whether the surgery is emergency or elective and whether the anesthesia to be used is general or local.

GENERAL ANESTHESIA

Elective Surgery

The patient scheduled for elective surgery should be allowed sufficient time to achieve the best possible general health and control of blood glucose before admission to the hospital. Complete evaluation of metabolic state and thorough assessment of diabetic complications, including renal and heart disease, is highly desirable before surgery.

The primary-care physician, surgeon, and anesthesiologist (preferably one experienced in diabetes management during surgery) should cooperate in preparing the diabetic patient for surgery. The anesthetic technique chosen should minimize disruption of metabolic control and, if possible, the operation should be scheduled for early morning to avoid prolonged fasting. This also makes it more likely that any postoperative metabolic care can be suitably provided.

In the past few years, an increasing number of authorities have advocated intravenous infusion of insulin rather than subcutaneous administration during the perioperative period. Intravenous infusion allows careful control of the amount and speed of insulin delivery and circumvents problems in the event of peripheral shutdown (e.g., hypotension, shock), which might occur during major surgery. For these reasons, intravenous insulin delivery is preferred during surgery. However, if the patient has stable pre-operative glucose control, the procedure is relatively minor, and recovery is expected to be rapid, then subcutaneous insulin administration may be a reasonable alternative.

Suggested guidelines for management of diabetic patients by use of intravenous insulin are found in Table 4.11. Guidelines for the subcutaneous route are in Table 4.12.

Emergency Surgery

In the event of emergency surgery requiring general anesthesia, there may not be sufficient time to optimally evaluate and stabilize the patient. Patients with diabetic ketoacidosis (DKA) who need emergency surgery represent a particular problem. In these patients, efforts should be made to delay surgery until the ketoacidosis is treated, even if not to complete resolution.

If surgery cannot be postponed, treatment of DKA should be initiated (as described in KETOACIDOSIS, pages 77–82) and continued throughout the operative and perioperative period. Once blood glucose level has fallen >300 mg/dl (>16.7 mM), insulin should be continued but at the rate described in Table 4.11.

Potassium should be checked frequently (every 1–2 h for the first 4 h and every 3–4 h thereafter). If potassium is normal or low with acidosis, intravenous potassium should be administered according to the algorithm described for ketoacidosis. These guidelines are similar to those described in KETOACIDOSIS.

LOCAL ANESTHESIA

Patients undergoing elective surgery with local anesthesia (e.g., dental work) generally should eat only after surgery, and surgery should preferably be scheduled as the first case to minimize duration of fasting. Insulin dose should be decreased on the morning of surgery. One approach is to give one-half to two-thirds of the customary dose of interme-

---

Table 4.11. Intravenous Insulin Regimen for Elective Surgery

The simplicity of this regimen and the ease of adjustment of insulin or glucose infusion rates have made it the preferred mode of insulin delivery during surgery.

Preoperative days
Attempt to obtain reasonable glycemic control (i.e., preprandial glucose concentrations >80 but <180 mg/dl [>4.4 but <10.0 mM]). If necessary, admit patient 2–3 days before surgery for this purpose. Most patients will require at least 2 injections of intermediate-acting insulin; many will require additional preprandial short-acting insulin. Insulin dose adjustments are generally based on preprandial glucose concentrations at 0800, 1200, 1800, and 2200.

Operative day
On the morning of surgery, keep patient NPO, omit usual subcutaneous insulin, and insert intravenous infusion line.

Start infusion of 5 g/h dextrose (D5W or D10W) with 2 meq/h KCl.

Administer insulin as follows:
- Begin with infusion of 1 U/h short-acting insulin.
- Evaluate blood glucose every 2–4 h before surgery, every hour during surgery, and every 2–4 h after surgery.
- Do not change infusion rate if blood glucose remains between 120 and 180 mg/dl (6.7–10.0 mM).
- Increase infusion rate by 0.5 U/h if blood glucose value is >180 mg/dl (>10.0 mM).
- Decrease infusion rate by 0.5 U/h if blood glucose value is <120 mg/dl (<6.7 mM).

Note: In children, the hourly rate of fluid infusion is adjusted to be consistent with daily maintenance fluid requirements of ~1500 ml/m^2 body surface area. Nevertheless, 1 U insulin/5 g glucose should be infused.

After surgery
When meals are resumed, discontinue intravenous insulin infusion and resume subcutaneous insulin as described in Table 4.12.

Table 4.12. Subcutaneous Insulin Regimen for Elective Surgery

Preoperative days
See Table 4.11.

Operative day
On the morning of surgery, keep patient NPO and adjust dose in the following manner. (The patient's basal insulin requirements continue during the perioperative period.)

Usual type of insulin	Morning of surgery
Intermediate acting	50–66% of usual dose
Short acting	Omit
Long acting (e.g., ultralente)	Usual dose
CSII	Usual basal coverage

Start an intravenous infusion of dextrose (D5W). In adults, set rate at ~100 ml/h. In children, the hourly rate is adjusted to be consistent with daily fluid requirements of ~1500 ml/m^2 body surface area.

During surgery

■ **Insulin**. Inject small amount of subcutaneous insulin if glucose is >200 mg/dl (>11.1 mM), according to the suggested algorithm below. In prepubertal children, halve these amounts.

Glucose		Insulin (U)
mg/dl	mM	
200–250	11.1–13.9	2-4
250–300	13.9–16.7	4-6
≥300	≥16.7	6-8

Give supplemental subcutaneous insulin only every 4 h. Decrease glucose infusion rate or begin insulin infusion at ~5–10 U/L D5W if blood glucose concentration continues to rise.

■ **Glucose**. Continue infusion of dextrose (D5W) at a rate of ~100 ml/h, or as appropriate for children. The following are regimens for treating low blood glucose.
■ If ≤80 mg/dl (≤4.4 mM), increase glucose infusion rate by 50%.
■ If ≤60 mg/dl (≤3.3 mM), or

■ If patient is symptomatic, give an intravenous bolus of glucose (~1 g/5- to 10- mg/dl (0.3- to 0.6-mM) increment in blood glucose desired); if fluid volume is a consideration, D10W or D20W may be used rather than D5W.

After surgery
■ **Insulin-glucose regimen**. Continue subcutaneous supplements and dextrose (D5W) infusion until oral feeding is resumed. If patient is NPO for several days, infuse sufficient glucose (150–200 g/day in adults; 2–4 g·kg^{-1}·day^{-1} in children) to meet minimal catabolic needs. Adjust the insulin infusion (initially ~10 U/L D5W) to prevent hyperglycemia or hypoglycemia.
■ **Transition to oral feeding**. If patient is able to eat and on a program that includes
  ■ **Prerandial short-acting insulin plus evening intermediate-acting insulin:** 30 min before a meal, inject sufficient short-acting insulin to cover ingested calories. If necessary, supplement with short-acting insulin according to the above algorithm. The meal should be available at the nursing station before the patient receives insulin. Give late-evening dose of intermediate-actinginsulin as usual.
  ■ **Intermediate-acting insulin only**: modify evening dose of intermediate-acting insulin in proportion to the number of calories consumed during the day.
  ■ **Long-acting or continuous subcutaneous insulin infusion:** continue customary basal dose of long-acting insulin or the basal rate of insulin infusion pump.

In all cases, monitor blood glucose every 4 h. Give supplements of insulin or glucose depending on SMBG results. When meals are fully tolerated, the presurgery insulin regimen can be reinstituted.

Succeeding postoperative days
Insulin dose will increase as the patient's calorie intake increases. Blood glucose measured before meals and at bedtime should be used to guide insulin dose adjustments.

diate-acting insulin or the full dose of long-acting insulin. Short-acting insulin should be omitted.

Glucose concentration should be measured before surgery. If it exceeds 240 mg/dl (>13.3 mM), a small amount of short-acting insulin should be given with an algorithm similar to that given in Table 4.12.

If glucose is <60 mg/dl (<3.3 mM) postoperatively, an intravenous bolus of glucose (~1 g for each 5- to 10-mg/dl [0.3- to 0.6-mM] increment in blood glucose desired) should be given or the patient allowed to eat or drink. Generally, the customary meal plan and insulin program may be continued postoperatively. This may require supplemental blood glucose monitoring with adjustments of insulin based on premeal blood glucose levels.

In the case of emergency surgery requiring a local anesthesia, every effort should be made to measure blood glucose concentration before surgery begins; the guidelines above should be followed.

CONCLUSION

Medical management of the diabetic patient requiring surgery must focus on provision of glucose and insulin in amounts to avoid hypoglycemia or hyperglycemia during and after surgery. Intravenous insulin and glucose at a rate providing ~1 U short-acting insulin for each 5 g glucose and frequent blood glucose monitoring will usually keep blood glucose levels between 120 and 250 mg/dl (6.7–13.9 mM). Major elective surgery in these patients is best performed in centers capable of integrating anesthetic, surgical, and medical care in a team approach.

BIBLIOGRAPHY

Gavin LA: Management of diabetes mellitus during surgery. *West J Med* 151:525–529, 1989

Gill GV, Alberti KGMM: The care of the diabetic patient during surgery. In *International Textbook of Diabetes Mellitus*. Alberti KGMM, DeFronzo RA, Keen, H, Zimmet P, Eds. Chichester, Wiley, 1992, p. 1173–83

Husband DJ, Thai AC, Alberti KGMM: Management of diabetes during surgery with glucose-insulin-potassium infusion. *Diabetic Med* 3:69–74, 1986

Pezzarossa A, Taddei F, Cimicchi MC, Rossini E, Contini S, Bonoro E, Gnudi A, Uggeri E: Perioperative management of diabetic subjects: subcutaneous versus intravenous insulin administration during glucose-potassium infusion. *Diabetes Care* 11:52–58, 1988

Walts LF, Miller J, Davidson MB, Brown J: Perioperative management of diabetes mellitus. *Anesthesiology* 55:104–109, 1981

Psychosocial Problems: Helping Patients Cope

Highlights
Psychosocial Problems:
Helping Patients Cope

DIAGNOSIS

Emotional distress is high at the time of diagnosis, but psychological equilibrium is generally reestablished within the 1st yr.

Intervention at diagnosis may improve adaptation, adherence, and metabolic control. Intervention strategies are suggested beginning on page 106.

MAINTAINING ADHERENCE

Over many years of diabetes, motivation to maintain optimal diabetes control may wane. Maintenance strategies include planning a workable diabetes regimen, improving patient/physician communication, and employing research-tested educational and behavioral strategies (Table 5.2).

COMPLICATIONS

Psychosocial factors should be suspected in the case of recurrent diabetic ketoacidosis.

Repeat episodes of severe hypoglycemia can have serious psychosocial consequences, which call for medical, educational, and family intervention.

When chronic complications begin, feelings of anger and guilt are common. A rehabilitation program that includes psychological counseling can help resolve the emotional reactions.

DEVELOPMENTAL CONSIDERATIONS

Although a diagnosis of diabetes during childhood is a devastating experience for parents and children, families are usually resilient and adapt to the demands of the regimen within the 1st yr.

Children's responsibilities for care should increase in tandem with cognitive and psychological development (Table 5.3). Children who take some responsibility for their diabetes care are generally more knowledgeable about their diabetes and are in better metabolic control. Caution should be exercised in forcing too much self-care too soon.

ADOLESCENTS

For adolescents, peer influences, together with family support and supervision, play an important role in adherence and glycemic control.

Many aspects of the treatment regimen are at odds with adolescent's normal drive for independence and peer acceptance.

ADULTS

Adults with diabetes must deal with a disease that often complicates their marriages and their attempts to establish a family and career and presents a financial burden as well.

OLDER ADULTS

The demands of the diabetes regimen may be especially burdensome for the elderly, who face other difficult life crises such as retirement, loss of physical function, living on a fixed income, the death of a spouse and/or friends, and their own mortality.

The goal is to provide support while safeguarding the patient's autonomy and independence as much as possible.

PSYCHIATRIC DISORDERS

The physician should recognize psychiatric illness in diabetic patients and refer them for treatment.

Psychopathology often goes undetected and untreated in patients with diabetes and other medical diseases.

Depression and anxiety disorders have been found to occur frequently in patients with diabetes.

Eating disorders should be suspected in young diabetic women with a history of unstable or poor metabolic control, recurrent ketoacidosis, or recurrent severe hypoglycemia, and in girls with growth retardation, pubertal delay, and/or amenorrhea.

STRESS

Results of numerous studies investigating the relationship between stress and blood glucose have been contradictory and inconclusive. Some show an association; some do not. Others show that patients may vary dramatically in their response to the same stressor.

Stress can indirectly affect blood glucose control by undermining adherence to the diabetes treatment regimen.

Psychosocial Problems: Helping Patients Cope

INTRODUCTION

Although insulin-dependent (type I) diabetes taxes the patient's psychosocial well-being, the converse is also true; psychosocial factors affect diabetes management. The unrelenting demands, inconveniences and frustrations of treatment, and threat of early disability or death put a tremendous strain on the diabetic patient and family. Patients must struggle continuously to achieve a balance between the demands of their everyday lives and those of their diabetes regimen. To help patients cope successfully with their diabetes in their real-life situations, the health-care team must consider the patient's daily schedule, lifestyle, and developmental stage when making diabetes management decisions and establishing treatment goals.

DIAGNOSIS

Psychological and emotional distress is high at the time of diagnosis (Table 5.1). Initial shock, denial, and anger often give way to mild depression and anxiety. Studies of newly diagnosed children and their families have found, however, that the initial reactions of both parents and children resolve rather quickly and psychological equilibrium is reestablished within the 1st yr. More extreme or long-lasting psychological reactions may indicate a need for referral to a mental health professional for evaluation and treatment.

Intervention at diagnosis or in the weeks after diagnosis may improve adaptation, prevent psychosocial maladjustment, and improve compliance and metabolic control. The health-care team can be a great help during this period by being accessible and sensitive to the patient's and family's need for information, even repeated several times. The following are suggestions for intervention aimed at facilitating adjustment and enhancing metabolic control.

■ It is essential that the patient's family is involved in the initial discussions and education of diabetes. Both parents in the case of a child, the patient's spouse, the adult children in the case of an elderly patient, or any significant others should be included. This is important given the wealth of research showing significant associations between related family factors and adherence. In addition to involving the family in diabetes education, the health-care team can strengthen support for the patient by encouraging family members to assist with diabetes tasks and responsibilities.

■ A comprehensive approach to diabetes education and management can be achieved if the physician assumes a leadership role in involving and coordinating the efforts of other members of the health-care team. Involvement of a nurse educator, a dietitian, a social worker, and/or a psychologist will ensure that the patient and family receive the education, dietary, and psychosocial support they need.

■ Self-management education with newly diagnosed diabetic children and their families in the months after diagnosis prevents deterioration in metabolic control during the first 2 yr after diagnosis of type I diabetes. Close follow-up by the health-care team in the weeks after the initial education will increase, reinforce, and clarify diabetes knowledge. Furthermore, emphasis on developing self-management strategies during these weeks appears to enhance adaptation and metabolic control. Self-management education includes reinforcement of accurate glucose monitoring and recording and the use of these data to understand blood glucose fluctuations and to make appropriate insulin and behavioral treatment changes. The goal is to help patients adopt a problem-solving approach to diabetes self-management. See also DIABETES SELF-MANAGEMENT EDUCATION, pages 21–30.

MAINTAINING ADHERENCE

There are high rates of relapse associated with attempts to change behaviors related to alcohol, drug addiction, smoking, and eating disorders. These stem, in part, from the lack of emphasis on the maintenance phase of treatment. Failures in diabetes management adherence and poor metabolic control are frequently the result of the same lack of attention to maintenance issues. The strategies listed in Table 5.2 may help facilitate long-term adherence.

DIABETES COMPLICATIONS

Short-Term Complications

Recurrent ketoacidosis is commonly the consequence of insulin omission that occurs because of psychosocial problems (e.g., financial stress, parental neglect, lack of family involvement, chronic family conflict, or eating disorders). Psychosocial factors should always be suspected in the case of recurrent ketoacidosis, and a psychiatric evaluation should be considered for these patients.

Severe Hypoglycemia

Most patients with well-controlled type I diabetes experience several mild low blood glucose reactions each month. In general, these mild reactions, although distracting and uncomfortable, do not pose a serious problem for the patient. Severe hypoglycemia, however, defined as an episode in which patients are unable to treat themselves, lose consciousness, and/or have seizures, can be frightening and may have serious neurologic and psychosocial consequences. The patient may become phobic about hypoglycemia and decide to maintain blood glucose values at unacceptably high levels. The family may also become

---

Table 5.1. Factors Causing Emotional Distress at Diagnosis

- Uncertainty about the outcome of the immediate situation
- Feelings of intense guilt and/or anger about the occurrence of diabetes
- Feelings of incompetence and helplessness about the responsibility for management of the illness
- Fears about future complications and early death
- Loss of valued life goals and aspirations because of illness
- Anxiety about planning for an uncertain future
- Recognition of the necessity for a permanent change in living pattern due to diabetes

Adapted from Hamburg BA, Inoff GE: Coping with predictable crises of diabetes. *Diabetes Care* 6:409–16, 1983

---

overly fearful, watchful, or angry, blaming the patient for the disturbing episodes. Patients who experience severe hypoglycemia at work may jeopardize their job or chances for advancement. Many patients with long-standing, well-controlled type I diabetes fail to recognize the early warning symptoms of hypoglycemia (hypoglycemia unawareness). These patients are at risk for repeated episodes of severe hypoglycemia and attendant medical and psychosocial consequences. Therefore, efforts should be made to prevent these episodes through reeducation and adjustments in the diabetes regimen (see HYPOGLYCEMIA, pages 85–86). The physician should discuss the patient's attitudes regarding hypoglycemia and help to establish safe blood glucose goals. The family or significant others should be trained to recognize early or subtle hypoglycemic signs and to be able to provide adequate prevention and treatment measures, including the administration of glucagon. If the family is angry and blames the patient, the health-care team will need to help the family understand the difficulty many patients have in recognizing and avoiding hypoglycemia. The family should also understand that the patient frequently cannot control his/her behavior during a severe low blood glucose reaction.

Table 5.2. Strategies to Improve and Maintain Adherence

The office
- Provide a convenient office location and facilities.
- Make appointment times as flexible as possible.
- Use appointment reminders.
- Schedule frequent appointments.

The health-care team
- Improve communication between patient and team members.
- Elicit patient expectations.
- Discuss expectations.
- Give specific instructions.
- Avoid jargon.
- Encourage questions and opinions from the patient.
- Encourage patient-focused interactions.

The regimen
- Involve the patient and family in treatment planning.
- Honor patient preferences and negotiate differences when planning the regimen and establishing treatment goals.
- Reduce the complexity and cost of the regimen when possible.
- Tailor the regimen to the patient's family lifestyle, culture, and finances.

Educational strategies
- Update diabetes knowledge to keep pace with developing technology and changing patient needs.
- Provide clearly written, easily understood instructions to reduce misunderstandings and forgetfulness.

Behavioral strategies
- Encourage personal responsibility and self-management approaches.
- Negotiate realistic glucose and behavioral goals to be achieved between clinic visits (written contracts make these agreements more concrete).
- Reinforce positive adherence behaviors and attainment of behavioral and glucose goals.
- Continue to encourage family involvement and the use of community support mechanisms.
- Help patients identify and plan ahead for situations that might result in a lapse in adherence.
- Analyze and help patients learn from adherence lapses.
- Help patients keep on track through follow-up phone calls, by responding to regularly mailed or faxed glucose records, and by using memory meters or glucose logs that allow the display of glucose trends and glucose averages over several weeks.

Long-Term Complications

Although most patients are aware of the possibility of long-term complications of diabetes, the detection of the first evidence of retinopathy, nephropathy, or neuropathy can be a devastating event. When the threat of a severe complication occurs, the patient and family must cope with the grief associated with the potential or actual loss of body function. Once again, the patient and family may experience feelings of shock, denial, and anger. Feelings of anger at the physician for "letting this happen" or guilt ("I should have taken better care of myself") are common. These feelings can be eased by emphasizing the positive steps that can still be taken to forestall or prevent serious problems. In more severe cases, the physician may need to refer a patient to a rehabilitation program that includes expert care and counseling by experienced health-care professionals. Support groups or contact with people who have successfully adapted to complications can provide useful information and role models and help patients maintain a hopeful outlook.

The physician and patient may be hesitant to broach the issue of sexual dysfunction—a common complication of diabetes in adults. It is critical to ask patients routinely about sexual function in a straightforward manner. Patients may be more likely to confide in the physician, or another member of the health-care team, if they know that sexual problems are common in diabetes and that a variety of treatment options are available.

DEVELOPMENTAL CONSIDERATIONS IN DIABETES MANAGEMENT

Children

Although a diagnosis of diabetes during childhood is a devastating experience for parents and children, families are usually resilient and adapt to the demands of the regimen within the 1st yr. Some of those demands, viewed from a developmental perspective, are outlined in Table 5.3.

Generally, children's responsibilities for care should increase in tandem with cognitive and psychological development. Children who take responsibility for their diabetes care are generally more knowledgeable about their diabetes and are in better metabolic control. When treating a school-age child, the health-care team should be alert for cognitive deficits that may interfere with drawing the correct amount of insulin, interpreting self-monitoring of blood glucose (SMBG) results accurately, or calculating food exchanges.

Self-esteem is built through mastery of the developmental tasks of childhood. Children feel good about themselves when they succeed in tasks such as toilet-training, getting dressed by themselves, doing well in their studies, making a goal in soccer, or helping with chores at home. Children with diabetes have more opportunities to build self-esteem when they learn to perform diabetes-related tasks. These may be as simple as setting up supplies for blood glucose tests or as advanced as calculating the correct dose and giving their own injections. This is especially true if parents, the health-care team, and others provide positive reinforcement for their

Table 5.3. Developmental Issues and Tasks in Children With Type I Diabetes

Infant (0–1 yr)	Differentiate hypoglycemic reactions from "normal" distress
	Parents are overwhelmed by demands of diabetes
	Identify and train trustworthy babysitters
Toddler (1–3 yr)	Differentiate misbehavior from hypoglycemia
	Expect dietary inconsistency as child begins to feed self
	Give child choices in food, injection, and fingerstick sites (avoid mealtime battles)
	Encourage child to report "funny" feelings (hypoglycemia)
	Let child begin to "help" with diabetes tasks
Preschool (3–6 yr)	Teach child to report hypoglycemia to adults in charge
	Teach child what to eat when "low"
	Reassure child who may view fingersticks and injections as punishment and/or become overly fearful of procedures
	Teach preschool teachers about diabetes
	Encourage child to participate in simple diabetes tasks
	Involve child in menu planning
School age (6–12 yr)	Teach all school personnel involved with child about diabetes
	Manage diabetes to minimize school absences
	Parents should foster age-appropriate independence
	Parents and child should learn to adjust insulin and regimen to encourage participation in social and sports events
	Encourage self-monitoring: recognize hypoglycemia; participate in meal planning; gradually learn to do own blood testing and injections: all activities to be supervised

Adapted from Schreiner B, Pontious S: Diabetes mellitus and the preschool child. In *Management of Diabetes Mellitus: Perspectives of Care Across the Life Span*. Haire-Joshu D, Ed. St. Louis, MO, Mosby Year Book, 1992, p. 362–98

achievements without forcing totally unsupervised behavior too early.

The Family

Diabetes impacts every aspect of family life and affects all family members. Research has shown that shared responsibility within the family relates to improved adherence and metabolic control. These results underscore the importance of defining diabetes tasks for each family member. Siblings, who commonly feel neglected or left out because of the extra attention given to the child with diabetes, may feel more involved if they are a part of the family's diabetes management effort. Fathers may be more likely to be involved if they, too, have clearly defined tasks. Full family involvement may help prevent over-involvement of the mother and overly close dependence between the mother and the child with diabetes.

Diabetes, School, and Peers

School entry is a difficult experience for most parents and children. It is even more traumatic for the parent and child with diabetes. Both must depend on teachers, who often are not knowledgeable about diabetes, to handle situations that could be life-threatening. The health-care team can help by providing diabetes literature and back-up for parents in their efforts to educate teachers, school nurses, and staff about diabetes.

An important goal of diabetes management during childhood is to prevent the diabetes regimen from disrupting the child's school experience. First, every effort should be made to ensure the child's safety at school. Hypoglycemia should be minimized, and school personnel should be trained to deal with specific diabetes-related problems such as meals, exercise, and signs of severe hypoglycemia. Second, the health-care team should work with parents, teachers, and school nurses to minimize absences and missed classes. Children may quickly learn to use their diabetes to avoid difficult school situations. Children who are frequently allowed to stay home for minor diabetes problems may fall behind in school and lose motivation to return to school.

During the elementary school years, peer relationships become increasingly important to children. This means that the health-care team must work with parents to ensure that children can attend birthday parties, slumber parties, and other normal childhood activities, even if this mean temporarily relaxing diabetes treatment goals or helping provide adjustments, i.e., extra insulin coverage for birthday cake.

ADOLESCENTS

Management of type I diabetes during the adolescent years is notoriously difficult. Note that many of the diabetes management principles presented in this section apply to other developmental stages as well.

For the young child with diabetes, successful adherence to the treatment regimen depends largely on parental interest, management skills, and other resources. For adolescents, peer influences, together with family support and supervision, play an increasingly important role in adherence and glycemic control. Many aspects of the treatment regimen are at odds with adolescent's normal drive for independence and peer acceptance. Experimentation with tobacco can lead to nicotine addiction. Experimentation with alcohol or other drugs can produce severe and life-threatening hypoglycemia. Adolescents may neglect monitoring, dietary considerations, insulin injections, and even visits to the clinic. These actions can have negative short- and long-term consequences. The health-care team can use various strategies to help the adolescent patient and family keep diabetes control within acceptable limits.

Understand the Scope of the Challenge

Almost all adolescents display characteristic behaviors and attitudes that reflect their drive for independence. Adolescents with diabetes are no exception. They undergo the same developmental process but with the added burden of diabetes. Hence, the health-care team should be prepared for a challenge.

However, do not assume that major difficulties are inevitable. There is no evidence that adolescents with diabetes suffer from serious psychological problems any more frequently than their nondiabetic peers. Many hormonal changes occur at puberty, some of which can adversely affect blood glucose levels. Puberty is associated with decreased sensitivity to insulin, and this may indicate an increase in insulin requirements. When the insulin dose is sufficient, an adolescent's problems in controlling diabetes during adolescence may be linked to social, family, or psychological factors; alcohol or drug use; or learning problems.

Family and Patient Factors

Because family routines overlap with the various aspects of the diabetic treatment regimen (i.e., timing and content of meals, need for monitoring and exercise), family factors and adherence to treatment are strongly interrelated. Adherence to treatment is better among adolescents if their families are characterized by lower levels of conflict, greater cohesiveness (i.e., family members interact more and are supportive of one another), and fewer negative interactions between parents and the adolescent.

Effective clinical interventions with diabetic adolescents and their families should target for change negative family interactions, especially those that focus on adherence. Because of the importance of self-care responsibilities in the management of diabetes, it is easy to blame and criticize the adolescent whenever blood glucose values are outside of a target range. Parents may need guidance in setting realistic expectations for their child's self-management behaviors and blood glucose levels and in dealing with unexpressed parental feelings of fear and guilt. Negative family interactions may have a negative impact on adherence.

Thus, educational interventions in adolescents should include parents and focus on the identification as well as use of measures that decrease diabetes-related conflicts and tensions in the family.

Health-Care Team Factors

In addition to acquiring an understanding of normal adolescent development, members of the health-care team should enjoy working with adolescents and show a genuine interest in them as individuals. If they cannot develop more than a superficial relationship, success in managing diabetes will be less likely. Likewise, clinicians must have confidence in their diabetes management skills. If not, referral to a specialist should be considered. The comments below should be applied to all members of the health-care team as appropriate.

Try to develop rapport. The health-care team should establish rapport with the patient but should not become part of the adolescent process itself. If any clinician is viewed by the adolescent negatively, as a surrogate parent, recommendations will be viewed by the adolescent in the same way as parental demands and may be rejected. Hence, clinicians must distance themselves from the parents during interactions with adolescents.

To avoid being viewed as a parental figure, the health-care team should make it clear to both the parents and the adolescent that they have responsibilities to each other. The clinician may agree or disagree with either the parents or the adolescent about different aspects of diabetes care. An attempt should be made to convince the adolescent that the clinician-patient relationship is not one between clinician and child, but one between clinician and young adult.

Be willing to compromise. Each member of the health-care team must be willing to compromise on almost all aspects of diabetes care and must clearly demonstrate respect for the adolescent's views. If a clinician becomes frustrated and angry when the adolescent does not adhere to the regimen, it will be difficult to retain the ability to influence the patient's self-care. It is not necessary to agree with the adolescent's views, but the clinician should at least listen to the patient and make an effort to accommodate the patient's wishes whenever possible.

Be consistent. An important factor known to affect adherence across all age groups is consistency in care-giving. The adolescent whose outpatient care is provided by any one of several different health-care team members with different management styles is not as likely to adhere to the regimen as is the patient seeing a health-care team with a consistent and predictable management style.

Individualized Treatment Regimens

The regimen should be as individually tailored as possible. Although complex regimens are less likely to be followed than simple regimens, individually negotiated regimens designed to meet the needs and requests of the patient should be encouraged. Adolescents, like adults, may be involved in many after-school activities and sports that demand a more complex regimen. The adolescent will be motivated to perform more frequent monitoring, take additional insulin injections, and to adhere to a specific meal plan if it is perceived that he or she can participate in desired activities or be granted special requests. Conversely, many adolescents can attain improved metabolic control with better adherence to a simplified regimen than little or no adherence to a more complex or demanding regimen. Negotiations regarding treatment regimens should be viewed by the adolescent and parents as attempts to accommodate the patient's treatment within lifestyle realities of adolescence.

Monitoring and Record-Keeping

Adolescents and their parents are frequently at odds about monitoring and record-keeping. At each clinic visit, the health-care team should negotiate with the adolescent on the type and frequency of SMBG as well as the kind of records to be maintained. The parents and the adolescent should be informed about various monitoring schedules and their advantages and disadvantages.

When discussing the importance of monitoring to an adolescent, the health-care team should emphasize that it is done primarily for the patient's benefit and not to placate or please the parents or physician. The adolescent should receive SMBG training (see MONITORING, pages 52–54). Adolescents will be more likely to monitor and record their results if these results are used to make management decisions and are perceived as increasing flexibility and safety while maintaining good metabolic control.

Periodically, the adolescent patient will refuse to monitor at all. The health-care team should not give up. Instead, renegotiate. If the adolescent is willing to perform one task, another can be added at a future office visit. This step-by-step approach often yields good results among adults as well as adolescents. One should stress to patients, however, that they need to resume monitoring if they become ill or are concerned about hypoglycemia.

Adolescents with diabetes commonly misrepresent glucose monitoring results. This is not surprising, given the many care demands, high parental and health-care team expectations, and the desire of the adolescent to be viewed as a "good patient." Misrepresentations can be of various types. One involves writing down results of tests never done. Another involves "editing" results so that undesirable values are "fixed," commonly by lowering high measurements. Yet another involves saving an old strip with a "good" reading and using this repeatedly to produce a desired pattern of glucose control. Misrepresentation should be suspected when the mean glucose values recorded are much lower than would be expected from a very high glycated hemoglobin level or when safe, round numbers appear to have been neatly recorded at the same time with the same pen.

After ruling out faulty measurement techniques and equipment and a form of hemoglobinopathy that would explain a higher-than-expected glycated hemoglobin level, misrepresentation of monitoring data for some secondary gain should be considered. When members of the health-care team suspect that home records misrepresent the facts, they should confront the adolescent with great care. Forcing a confession seldom serves a useful purpose. The health-care team should tell the patient that the blood glucose records are inconsistent with the glycated hemoglobin and, after ruling out other explanations for this discrepancy, urge the patient to be as accurate as possible in reporting blood glucose values. At the same time, the adolescent should be praised for testing and recording, even if blood glucose values are elevated. Also, they should be praised, not chastised, for leaving tests not done as blanks rather than filling them with fabricated values. No accusations should be made, and a problem-solving approach should be sought. This nonjudgmental approach may provide a good model for the parents, who should be encouraged not to punish the adolescent for having high but accurate glucose monitoring results. The health-care team should also remind parents that other adolescents with diabetes (and even adults) have problems adhering to the treatment regimen.

ADULTS

Marriage, family, employment, and finances are four major aspects of adulthood. Adults with diabetes must deal with a disease that often complicates their marriages, their attempts to establish a family and career, and presents a financial burden as well.

The health-care team can help get a patient's marriage off to a realistic start by arranging a meeting with the spouse-to-be to answer questions and provide information about diabetes, especially about the management of diabetes crises and the importance of supporting adherence to the treatment regimen. Family planning counseling will provide crucial information as the couple decides whether and/or when to have a child. Both partners should understand the risks of pregnancy for the woman with

diabetes and the need for optimal metabolic control at the time of conception (see PREGNANCY, pages 90–91).

The health-care team should be able to help patients in many other ways during the adult years. They can offer education and counsel when misunderstandings and conflicts arise in a marriage because of diabetes. They can refer patients to community, state, and federal programs to help with financial problems. They can educate and reassure children who worry about their parents' diabetes. Physicians can work with patients to match the regimen to the realities of the job and consult with employers if problems with diabetes management threaten a patient's job.

OLDER ADULTS

Due to increased survival rates, there is a growing number of older adults with type I diabetes. In addition, there is an increasing number of older patients with type II diabetes who require insulin.

Many older people are active and functional and may wish to increase rather than decrease the intensity of their diabetes care. Retired people may have more time and resources to devote to diabetes self-care skills. Because of the availability of Medicare coverage, older people may have greater access to health services and be able to afford to participate more actively in their care.

However, the demands of the diabetes regimen may be especially burdensome for some elderly, especially those who face other difficult life crises such as retirement, loss of physical function, living on a fixed income, the death of a spouse and/or friends, and their own mortality. It may be more difficult to keep physician appointments and purchase supplies because of transportation problems and financial limitations. The health-care team should be aware that errors in insulin administration and blood testing may be due to failing eyesight or poor coordination. Older patients are more likely to be forgetful and to become confused by new information. It is essential for the health-care team to carefully assess each older patient to identify and address these potential barriers to sound diabetes care.

Inevitably, there are changes in social support as one ages. Those who have helped in the past may no longer be able or available to do so. Social support is important to the health and well-being of older adults, but its role will vary by sex, race, marital status, and illness characteristics. Careful assessment will help to identify support people and to specify the type of help needed. The goal is to provide support while safeguarding the patient's autonomy and independence as much as possible. Home-care agencies and special programs, such as Meals-on-Wheels, are often helpful.

As emphasized for other age-groups, the relationships between the health-care team and patient will influence patient adherence. Patients who are satisfied with their team are more likely to adhere to their diabetes care plan. However, older adults are less likely than other age-groups to express dissatisfaction directly to the provider. Therefore, it is even more essential to encourage open communication with this group by asking and responding to questions and by taking time to show concern and discuss problems.

PSYCHIATRIC DISORDERS AND DIABETES

It is important that the physician recognize psychiatric disorders in patients with diabetes and refer these patients for evaluation and counseling. In studies investigating the degree to which nonpsychiatric physicians recognize and treat depression in patients with diabetes, depression was recognized and treated in fewer than one-third of patients diagnosed as clinically depressed using DSM-III criteria. These results are consistent with previous studies showing that psychopathology frequently goes undetected and untreated in patients with a chronic medical problem. Some physicians mistakenly view psychiatric symptoms, especially those of depression and anxiety, as expected or even normal in people coping with an illness as serious and difficult to treat as diabetes. Unfortunately, when psychiatric symptoms are seen as the norm, therapeutic intervention may not be recommended, and the patient will continue to suffer psychological distress. This situation is especially disturbing in light of the high prevalence of depression and anxiety in adults with diabetes and the availability of effective treatment options for the management of depression.

Eating disorders are common in young women with type I diabetes and are associated with poor metabolic control, poor adherence to the diabetic regimen, and more severe complications. DSM-IIIR diagnostic criteria for anorexia nervosa include weight loss and maintenance of body weight 15% below norm, impaired body image, intense fear of weight gain, and absence of menses. The DSM-IIIR diagnostic criteria for bulimia nervosa include recurrent episodes of binge-eating, feelings of loss of control over eating during binges, frequent self-induced vomiting and/or laxative use, and overconcern with body image and weight.

Many young people with type I diabetes may have eating disturbances that compromise their diabetes control yet do not meet stringent DSM-IIIR diagnostic criteria. The seriousness of these subclinical cases should not be underestimated because they can result in short- and long-term metabolic complications. Eating disorders, clinical and subclinical, should be suspected in young women with persistently unstable or poor metabolic control, recurrent ketoacidosis resulting from insulin omission to induce glycosuria and weight loss, or recurrent severe hypoglycemia due to food restriction while continuing insulin and in girls with growth retardation and pubertal delay. These patients may require referral to an experienced mental health professional for psychological evaluation and treatment if an explanation for their problems is not found.

STRESS AND DIABETES

Although physicians and patients have long observed a relationship between stress and blood glucose levels, the results of numerous studies attempting to define this relationship have resulted in contradictory results. Some studies have shown an association between stress and hyperglycemia, whereas others have not. In some studies, this relationship has been idiosyncratic, with patients varying dramatically in their glucose response to the same stressor.

Stress can also have indirect effects on diabetes. Patients under stress may be less able to follow their diabetes regimen, may give a low priority to their diabetes care, or may respond to the stress by overeating or increasing their use of alcohol or illicit drugs. The physician should explore these possible explanations for poor metabolic control. Some patients can learn to cope with stress management counseling or relaxation training.

BIBLIOGRAPHY

Anderson BJ, Auslander WF, Jung KC, Miller JP, Santiago JV; Assessing family sharing of diabetes responsibilities. *J Pediatr Psychol* 15: 477–92, 1990

Connell CM, Fisher EB, Houston CA: Relationships among social support, diabetes outcomes and morale for older men and women. *J Aging Health* 4:77–100, 1992

Delamater A, Bubb J, David SG, Smith JA, Schmidt L, White NH, Santiago JV: Randomized prospective study of self-management training with newly diagnosed diabetic children. *Diabetes Care* 13:492–98, 1990

Eraker SA, Kirsch JP, Becker MH: Understanding and improving patient compliance. *Ann Intern Med* 100:258–68, 1984

Jacobson AM, Hanser ST, Wolfsdorf JI, Houlihan J, Milley JE, Herskowitz RD, Werthieb D, Watt E: Psychological predictors of compliance in children with recent onset of diabetes mellitus. *J Pediatr* 108: 805–11, 1987

Johnson SB: Compliance and control in insulin-dependent diabetes: does behavior really make a difference? In *Perspectives in Behavioral Medicine: Stress and Disease Processes.* Schneiderman N, McCabe P, Baum A, Eds, Hillsdale, NJ, Erlbaum, 1992, p. 275–97

Johnson SB, Freund A, Silverstein J, Hansen CA, Malone J: Adherence-health status relationships in childhood diabetes. *Health Psychol* 9:606–31, 1990

Johnson SB, Silverstein J, Rosenbloom A, Carter R, Cunningham W: Assessing daily management of childhood diabetes. *Health Psychol* 5:545–64, 1986

Kovacs J, Brent D, Steinberg TF, Paulauskas S, Reid J: Children's self-report of psychologic adjustment and coping strategies during first year of insulin-dependent diabetes mellitus. *Diabetes Care* 9:472–79, 1986

La Greca AM, Follansbee D, Skyler JS: Developmental and behavioral aspects of diabetes management in youngsters. *Children's Health Care* 19:132–39, 1990

LaGreca AM, Skyler JS: Psychosocial issues in IDDM: a multivariate framework. In *Stress Coping and Disease.* McCabe P, Schneiderman N, Field T, Skyler JS, Eds. Hillsdale, NJ, Erlbaum, 1991, p. 169–90

Lustman PJ, Griffith LS, Couse RE, Cryer PE: Psychiatric illness in diabetes mellitus. *J Nerv Ment Dis* 174:736–42, 1986

Lustman PJ, Harper GW: Nonpsychiatric physicians' identification and treatment of depression in patients with diabetes. *Comp Psychiatry* 28:22–27, 1987

Pontious S, Tesno B: Diabetes mellitus and the school-age child. In *Management of Diabetes Mellitus: Perspectives of Care Across the Life Span.* Haire-Joshu D, Ed. St. Louis, MO, Mosby Year Book, 1992, p. 399–440

Rodin M, Daneman D: Eating disorders and IDDM. *Diabetes Care* 15:1402–12, 1992

Surwit RW, Schneider MS, Feinglos MN: Stress and diabetes. *Diabetes Care* 15:141–42, 1992

Complications

Highlights

Highlights
Complications

RETINOPATHY

Retinopathy in patients with type I diabetes rarely occurs before the 5th yr of the disease.

The clinician should evaluate the retinas of diabetic patients with the direct ophthalmoscope annually and when indicated by symptoms or previous findings. Indications for ophthalmological referral are described in Table 6.1.

High-risk characteristics of proliferative retinopathy greatly increase the risk of blindness and include
■ new vessels on the disk (NVD) greater than ~25% of the optic disk area,
■ any NVD with preretinal or vitreous hemorrhage, and
■ new vessels elsewhere ≥50% of the disk area (totaled for the entire retina) with preretinal or vitreous hemorrhage.
When high-risk characteristics are present, photocoagulation therapy is mandatory.

Lesions typical of background or nonproliferative retinopathy, preproliferative retinopathy, proliferative retinopathy, and macular edema are described on pages 120–121.

Treatment for diabetic retinopathy can be highly effective in preserving or salvaging vision. Treatment modalities include
■ panretinal photocoagulation,
■ focal laser photocoagulation, and
■ vitrectomy.

Medical therapies are discussed on pages 124–125.

NEPHROPATHY

Epidemiologic studies have shown that up to 30–40% of patients affected with type I diabetes will eventually develop end-stage renal failure and require dialysis.

Possible mechanisms by which diabetes damages the kidney are discussed on page 128. Elevated blood glucose, a genetic propensity, elevated blood pressure, and abnormal glomerular hemodynamics have been proposed.

Renal function should be monitored regularly in all patients with type I diabetes (Table 6.2).

Patients with diabetes and persistent microalbuminuria are at a higher risk for developing renal insufficiency and may benefit from more intensive follow-up and therapy.

The management of diabetic nephropathy is largely preventive and supportive. It consists of minimizing factors that are known to accelerate the natural progression of renal disease or that may otherwise jeopardize the kidney and of appropriately responding to changing insulin needs (Tables 6.3 and 6.4).

If end-stage renal failure ensues, two options are available: dialysis and kidney transplantation.

NEUROPATHY

Diabetic neuropathy is classified into a set of discrete clinical syndromes, each with a characteristic presentation and clinical course (Table 6.5). The syndromes overlap clinically and frequently occur simultaneously.

Distal symmetrical polyneuropathy is the most common form of diabetic neuropathy.

Patients with chronic, unrecognized neuropathy may present with late complications, e.g., foot ulceration, foreign objects embedded in the foot, unrecognized trauma to the extremities, or neuroarthropathy (Charcot's joints). All of these conditions are avoidable with proper early diagnosis of neuropathy and institution of appropriate foot care.

Treatment for diabetic distal symmetric polyneuropathy is symptomatic, palliative, and supportive, with primary emphasis on preventing the late complications.

Persistent and severely painful neuropathy has been treated with various drugs, including standard analgesics and drugs normally used to treat pain in other conditions. Narcotics should be avoided except in the most extreme cases.

Although autonomic neuropathy produces diffuse subclinical dysfunction, autonomic symptoms are usually confined to one or two organ systems, producing the discrete autonomic syndromes listed in Table 6.8.

Erectile impotence in diabetic men may be psychogenic, endocrine, vascular, drug or stress related, or neuropathic.

Other dysfunctions related to autonomic neuropathy include diabetic cystopathy and hypoglycemic unawareness.

Mononeuropathies comprise neural deficits corresponding to the distribution of single or multiple peripheral nerves.

MACROVASCULAR COMPLICATIONS

Coronary heart disease, peripheral vascular disease, and cerebrovascular disease are more common, tend to occur at an earlier age, and are more extensive and severe in people with diabetes.

Physicians should systematically assess patients for risk factors for atherosclerotic cardiovascular disease, question them about symptoms, and be alert for signs of atherosclerosis.

A program for modifying risk factors should be started if appropriate.

Guidelines for treatment of cerebrovascular disease, coronary heart disease, and peripheral vascular disease appear on pages 143–144.

LIMITED JOINT MOBILITY

Limited joint mobility (LJM) is a potentially important clinical marker for diabetes complications such as retinopathy, nephropathy, neuropathy, and other disorders. Glycation of tissue proteins may be responsible for LJM.

LJM may occur in children or adults, is painless, and can cause some disability. It is marked by a sclerodermalike stiffness of the skin and joints; ultimately, all joints may be affected.

Patients found to have LJM should be examined carefully for complications, e.g., retinopathy, nephropathy, neuropathy, hypertension, and hepatomegaly.

GROWTH

Subtle abnormalities of growth and development affect 5–10% of youngsters with type I diabetes and usually result from inadequate metabolic control.

Signs of growth abnormalities include a lag in height or weight or a falling away from the patient's previously established growth curves (Figure 6.11).

Children most likely to be affected are those with the earliest onset of diabetes and the worst glycemic control. Boys are 2–3 times more likely to be affected than girls.

To detect growth abnormalities, the physician should regularly plot height and weight on standard growth charts. Other growth-impairing conditions should be considered in assessing growth abnormalities (Figure 6.12).

Retinopathy

INTRODUCTION

Diabetic retinopathy is one of the four most common causes of blindness in the United States and is a major cause of visual disability. Several surveys suggest that a person with diabetes has a 5–10% chance of becoming legally blind and that this risk is greater in people with type I versus type II diabetes.

Retinopathy in patients with type I diabetes rarely occurs before the 5th yr of the disease, but retinopathy detected by fundus photography reaches a prevalence of 50% by the 10th yr. By the 15th yr, up to 50% of patients have proliferative retinopathy, in which new blood vessels develop from the retinal circulation, with a substantial risk of severe hemorrhage and traction detachment of the retina. After 20 yr duration of diabetes, >90% of patients will have retinopathy. Retinopathy rarely occurs before the onset of puberty, even in patients with diabetes >5 yr. The hormonal changes of puberty seem to exert an accelerating influence on the development of retinopathy.

EYE EXAMINATION

Because diabetic retinopathy appears primarily in the posterior retina within a few optic disk diameters of the optic nerve head (disk) and the macula, most lesions are readily seen by the nonophthalmologist with the monocular direct ophthalmoscope. Every physician should learn how to use this instrument.

Visualization of the retina is enhanced by dilating the pupils, which is easily accomplished in most patients with 1 drop each of 2.5% phenylephrine hydrochloride and 1% tropicamide. This procedure carries little risk in younger people. Angle-closure glaucoma, a major complication, is a rare disorder in any age group and is virtually nonexistent before age 40 yr. Blurred near vision and sensitivity to bright lights (requiring the use of dark glasses) are temporary inconveniences, lasting only a few hours.

This examination is not an adequate substitute for an evaluation by a qualified eye doctor. The appropriate role for a nondilated-pupil, single-field screening fundus photograph has not yet been defined.

CLINICAL FINDINGS IN DIABETIC RETINOPATHY

Background or Nonproliferative Retinopathy

The earliest lesion visible through the ophthalmoscope is the microaneurysm, a pouchlike dilation of a terminal capillary. Ophthalmoscopically, microaneurysms look like tiny red dots. Dot hemorrhages may be indistinguishable from microaneurysms unless specialized techniques such as fluorescein angiography are used, but blot hemorrhages are easily recognized because they are larger (Figure 6.1). Hard exudates are another common feature of background (nonproliferative) retinopathy. Background retinopathy does not cause visual symptoms unless it is associated with macular edema.

Preproliferative Retinopathy

Multiple clustered blot hemorrhages suggest progression to the preproliferative (or severe nonproliferative) stage because they indicate that substantial portions of the capillary circulation have become nonfunctional, i.e., are nonperfused. It is believed that new blood vessels are formed as a result of the retina's great metabolic need for oxygen and other nutrients supplied by the bloodstream. According to this hypothesis, areas of retinal nonperfusion call forth an angiogenic response that stimulates the growth of abnormal new blood vessels.

Veins may appear dilated, tortuous, and irregular in caliber. Intraretinal microvascular abnormalities (IRMAs) are other signs of preproliferative retinopathy. These small loops of fine vessels usually extend from a major artery or vein and probably represent early new-vessel formation within the retina. Fluffy white lesions, commonly referred to as cotton-wool spots, were formerly associated with preproliferative retinopathy. Evidence suggests that

120

these lesions, when they appear alone, may not be poor prognostic indicators.

Proliferative Retinopathy

Proliferative diabetic retinopathy involves the formation of new blood vessels, extending from within the retinal substance onto the inner surface of the retina or into the vitreous cavity. These commonly occur on the optic nerve head, where they are called new vessels on the disk (NVD) (Figure 6.2), or elsewhere in the retina, usually extending from major vessels, where they are called new vessels elsewhere (NVE). New vessels are fragile and carry a substantial risk of rupture with hemorrhage or of producing retinal detachment from the tractional forces exerted by the accompanying strands of fibrous tissue on the thin, tissue-paper–like retina.

Certain findings were defined as high-risk characteristics (HRCs) by the national Diabetic Retinopathy Study (DRS), a large-scale, randomized, controlled, clinical trial completed in 1981. The presence of HRC increases an eye's risk of blindness (<5/200 vision) to 30–50% within 3–5 yr of detection if appropriate treatment is not given. High-risk characteristics include
■ NVD greater than ~25% of the optic disk area,
■ any NVD with preretinal or vitreous hemorrhage, and
■ NVE ≥50% of the disk area (totaled for the entire retina) with preretinal or vitreous hemorrhage (Figure 6.3). When HRCs are present, photocoagulation therapy is mandatory.

Diabetic Macular Edema

Macular edema involves thickening of the central portion of the retina, the macula, which occupies an area of ~5 disk diameters just temporal to the optic nerve head (Figure 6.4). Visual acuity is decreased in this condition, particularly when the center of the macula (the fovea centralis) is involved. Macular edema is difficult to diagnose with the direct ophthalmoscope because the monocular viewing system of this instrument does not allow the stereoscopic vision neces-sary to determine retinal thickening. However, the presence of hard lipid exudates—yellowish-white, often glistening deposits of round or irregular shape lying within the retina, usually in the macular region—strongly suggests macular edema. This is particularly true if the exudates assume a ring-shaped, or circinate, configuration. The features of clinically significant macular edema are
■ retinal thickening near the macular center,
■ hard exudates near the macular center and adjacent retinal thickening, and
■ retinal thickening >1 disk diameter in size and within 1 disk diameter of the macular center.

Glaucoma

Sometimes, in far-advanced (usually proliferative) diabetic retinopathy, new vessels may also form on the surface of the iris and extend into the "angle" of the anterior chamber of the eye, where the cornea and iris come together (Figures 6.5–6.8). Here, fibrous scar tissue extending from the new vessels may block the outflow of aqueous humor from the eye, causing a rise in intraocular pressure (neovascular glaucoma), severe pain, and loss of vision.

EVALUATION

The clinician should evaluate the retinas of diabetic patients with the direct ophthalmoscope annually and when indicated by symptoms or previous findings.

Patients with type I diabetes should have an annual detailed ocular examination after 5 yr duration of diabetes; the examination need not be done before puberty unless the patient has eye symptoms or evidence of other complications of diabetes. The examination should be done by an experienced eye-care specialist and should include
■ determination of visual acuity of each eye,
■ refraction, if visual acuity is impaired,
■ gross external examination of the eyes,
■ evaluation of ocular motility,

Figure 6.1. Background or Nonproliferative Diabetic Retinopathy

Fundus of patient's left eye is shown, with optic nerve head at far left and center of macula appearing as darker zone at center. Note scattered microaneurysm and dot hemorrhages and minimal amount of lipid to right of (temporal to) center of macula.

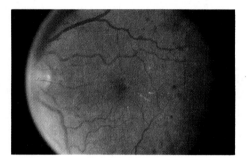

Figure 6.2. Neovascularization of Disk

Neovascularization of this extent (>33% of the disk area) is one of the high-risk characteristics for progression to severe blindness during next 3 yr. *White marks* surrounding optic disk at *right* are laser burns, placed in pattern used for panretinal photocoagulation.

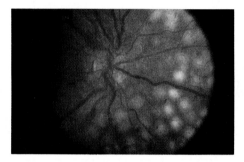

Figure 6.3. Preretinal Hemorrhage

Layered out between posterior face of vitreous gel and inner surface of retina, hemorrhage forms typical boat-shaped configuration. Preretinal hemorrhages may assume other shapes as well. Compact form of hemorrhage, its sharply defined borders, and its location in front of retinal vessels indicate that this is a preretinal not intraretinal hemorrhage. Preretinal or vitreous hemorrhages strongly suggest presence of neovascularization.

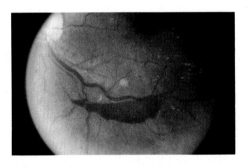

Figure 6.4. Diabetic Macular Edema

Macular region of right eye is shown. There is much lipid, most of which forms rings (circinate retinopathy). Lipid does not yet involve center of macula. In this monocular view, thickening (edema) of retina cannot be appreciated, especially in centers of lipid rings, but this would be evident by stereoscopic ophthalmoscopy or photographs.

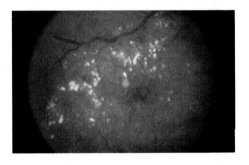

■ examination of the eyes by slit-lamp biomicroscopy,
■ examination of the retina with monocular direct and binocular indirect ophthalmoscopy after dilation of the pupils,
■ slit-lamp ophthalmoscopy to exclude macular edema, and

■ in adult patients, measurement of intraocular pressures.

Some examinations should be carried out only for specific indications. These include retinal photography, which is used to document special lesions, and intravenous fluorescein angiography. During this test, a fluorescent dye is

Figure 6.5. Preproliferative or Severe Nonproliferative Diabetic Retinopathy

Note markedly dilated and irregular veins. Beaded vein extending from center to 11-o'clock border of photograph looks like string of sausages. There are multiple blot hemorrhages and 2 cotton-wool spots just below major vein in *center*. Fan-shaped tuft of fine vessels just above major vein (*right center*) may represent early neovascularization. Round, bright white spot above major vein (*left center*) is photographic artifact.

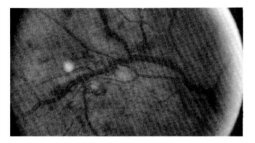

Figure 6.7. Proliferative Diabetic Retinopathy

Extensive fibrogial proliferation extends from optic disk, which is dimly seen in center. Retinal vessels are bent at right angles by traction from proliferation. Retina is partly detached, with severe loss of vision.

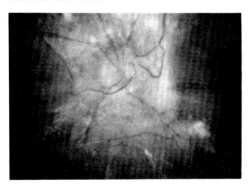

Figure 6.6. Proliferative Diabetic Retinopathy

Long, fine sprigs of flat neovascularizastion elsewhere (i.e., not on optic disk; also called NVE) arise in fan shape from major vein in *center*. Blot hemorrhages are in *upper left*.

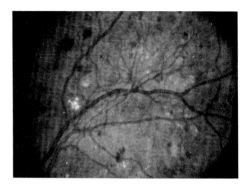

Figure 6.8. Neovascularization of Iris

This occurs in far-advanced usually proliferative diabetic retinopathy. Blood vessels are usually not visible on surface of iris, and extensive branching vessels of thick caliber, visible to left of pupil, are highly abnormal. They often grow to iris periphery, into anterior chamber angle, which they occlude by accompanying tough, fibrous tissue and by hemorrhage and scar formation between root of iris and inner surface of cornea. This produces extreme elevation of intraocular pressure, pain, and blindness. Pupil is irregular partly by contraction because of fibrous tissue and partly because of formation of posterior synechiae or scars between pupillary border of iris and underlying ocular lens.

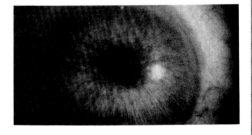

injected into the antecubital vein, and rapid-sequence photography of the retinal circulation is carried out with special colored filters in front of the photoflash unit and in front of the film plane of the camera. Both eyes are typically evaluated at a single injection sequence; it is not necessary to perform two separate angiograms to evaluate each eye individually.

Fluorescein angiography is useful clinically to plan photocoagulation treatment for macular edema. Although it is more sensitive than ophthalmoscopy or

Table 6.1. Guidelines for Care

Routine care by physician
- Examine retina with direct ophthalmoscope annually and when indicated by symptoms or previous findings

Referral to eye-care specialist
- Examine retinas through dilated pupils once a year (this need not be done before puberty unless the patient has eye symptoms or other complications of diabetes)

Referral to ophthalmologist
- At the beginning of pregnancy or if planning pregnancy within 12 mo
- Immediate referral is mandatory (preferably to an ophthalmologist specializing in retinal disease) if any of the following are present:
  - New vessels on the disk (NVD) greater than ~25% of the optic disk area
  - Any NVD with preretinal or vitreous hemorrhage
  - New vessels elsewhere (NVE) ≥50% of the disk area with preretinal or vitreous hemorrhage
- Macular edema (suggested by hard exudates within the macula)
- Reduced vision from any cause
- Immediate referral is strongly urged when the following are present:
  - Proliferative retinopathy without high-risk characteristics
    - Preproliferative retinopathy with
      - dilated irregular veins
      - multiple dot and blot hemorrhages
      - intraretinal microvascular abnormalities

color photography for detecting very early lesions of retinopathy, the minute lesions detected are rarely critical for making decisions regarding treatment. Therefore, intravenous fluorescein angiography should not be used as a screening test in the annual ocular examination of diabetic patients. Guidelines for care and referral are described in Table 6.1.

TREATMENT

Clinicians should always refer patients for treatment of retinopathy to an ophthalmologist, preferably one who is an expert in retinal disease. If laser treatment (described below) has been recommended, the clinician should check that the treatment has been implemented and that the patient maintains the recommended follow-up.

Photocoagulation

Panretinal Photocoagulation
The principle method used to treat diabetic retinopathy is by argon laser or xenon light photocoagulation. For patients with proliferative retinopathy and HRCs, panretinal photocoagulation with the laser is standard therapy, based on DRS results.

In this procedure, a series of 1200–1600 (or sometimes more) laser burns, 500 μm in diameter and spaced one-half burn diameter apart, are placed throughout the midperipheral retina, avoiding the macular region. The DRS demonstrated that this procedure reduced the rate of progression to blindness by 50% in eyes with HRCs over a 5-yr follow-up period.

Many eyes with proliferative retinopathy short of HRCs or with preproliferative retinopathy are also receiving panretinal photocoagulation, but the efficacy of this treatment is not as dramatic. The value of panretinal photocoagulation (or of "mild" panretinal photocoagulation, in which 450–650 burns are placed around the retina, with much wider spacing than in the standard treatment protocol) in these circumstances was evaluated in the Early Treatment Diabetic Retinopathy Study (ETDRS), another large-scale randomized, controlled, clinical trial. Panretinal photocoagulation also appears to reduce the risk of neovascular glaucoma in eyes with severe retinopathy.

Focal Laser Photocoagulation
Diabetic macular edema is currently treated by focal laser photocoagulation. With this technique, leaking microaneurysm and other vascular abnormalities in the macular region, determined by fluorescein angiography, are treated by direct application of small (50- to 100-μm) laser burns. The ETDRS recently showed that this treatment reduced the rate of visual loss from diabetic macular edema by 50% over a 3-yr follow-up

period. Photocoagulation is of no benefit for mild or moderate background retinopathy without macular edema.

Vitrectomy

Vitrectomy is a surgical procedure used to *1)* remove vitreous humor filled with blood, *2)* cut fibrous traction bands, *3)* peel contractile fibrous membranes from the inner retinal surface, and *4)* repair some types of complex retinal detachments. It is particularly effective in certain cases of advanced proliferative diabetic retinopathy. Although it can often restore useful vision to eyes that would otherwise be blind, vitrectomy is usually used only in severely diseased eyes, and recovery to near-normal vision after this surgery is the exception not the rule.

Medical Therapy

It is important to maintain normal blood pressure levels in diabetic patients with retinopathy because diabetic retinopathy progresses more rapidly in patients with uncontrolled hypertension than in those whose blood pressure is normal.

Therapies Under Evaluation

Other medical treatments for diabetic retinopathy have been evaluated.
- Aspirin (650 mg/day) was tested in the ETDRS because it inhibits platelet aggregation. Platelet microthrombi have been proposed as a factor in the cause of diabetic retinopathy. Aspirin was shown to be of no benefit or risk for retinopathy in this study.
- There is some evidence from animal experiments that a class of drugs called aldose reductase inhibitors is useful in preventing or reducing the progression of diabetic retinopathy. By inhibiting aldose reductase, these drugs prevent the enzymatic conversion of glucose to sorbitol, a reaction that is augmented in hyperglycemic states and may result in damage to certain highly susceptible cells, possibly including those of retinal blood vessels. Several short-term clinical trials have shown limited or no benefit of these investigational drugs in treating retinopathy. Longer trials are in process.

CONCLUSION

Diabetic retinopathy is a common complication of long-term diabetes mellitus that ranks as a leading cause of blindness and visual disability. Although current treatment strategies cannot totally prevent or cure this complication, there is significant evidence that they can substantially retard its progression when used appropriately and at the right time. Accordingly, careful evaluation of the ocular fundus of diabetic patients by the primary-care physician, with periodic referral to an eye doctor, is a standard of care for all patients with diabetes mellitus. In the Diabetes Control and Complications Trial (DCCT), intensively treated patients with preexisting mild to moderate retinopathy showed a 50% reduced risk of progressing to proliferative retinopathy or macular edema requiring photocoagulation.

BIBLIOGRAPHY

DCCT Research Group: The effect of intensive treatment of diabetes on the development and progression of long-term complications in insulin-dependent diabetes mellitus. *N Engl J Med* 329:977–86, 1993

Diabetic Retinopathy Study Research Group: Photocoagulation treatment of proliferative diabetic retinopathy: clinical application of Diabetic Retinopathy Study (DRS) findings. *Ophthalmology* 88:583–600, 1981

Diabetic Retinopathy Vitrectomy Study Research Group: Early vitrectomy for severe vitreous hemorrhage in diabetic retinopathy. *Arch Ophthalmol* 103:1644–52, 1985

Early Treatment Diabetic Retinopathy Study Research Group: Treatment techniques and clinical guidelines for photocoagulation of diabetic macular edema. *Ophthalmology* 94:761–74, 1987

Frank RN: On the pathogenesis of diabetic retinopathy. *Ophthalmology* 91:626–34, 1984

Klein R, Klein BEK, Moss SE, Davis MD, DeMets DL: The Wisconsin epidemiology study of diabetic retinopathy. II. Prevalence and risk of diabetic retinopathy when age at diagnosis is less than 30 yr. *Arch Ophthalmol* 102:520–26, 1984

Nephropathy

INTRODUCTION

In the past, epidemiologic studies have shown consistently that 30–40% of patients affected with type I diabetes will eventually develop end-stage renal failure and require dialysis. About one in every four individuals starting dialysis in the United States has diabetes, and almost half of these have type I diabetes. Recent evidence suggests that the frequency of nephropathy may be decreasing with the use of more effective diabetes treatment and antihypertensive therapy.

CLINICAL SYNDROME

In its fully established form, diabetic nephropathy is a distinct clinical entity characterized by proteinuria, hypertension, edema, and renal insufficiency, and it occurs in patients with long-standing (usually >10 yr) diabetes. The most consistent finding is proteinuria, which may be accompanied by hypoalbuminemia and dyslipidemia in its most severe forms (nephrotic syndrome).

Histopathologic Changes

Three classes of renal histopathologic changes characterize diabetic nephropathy: 1) glomerulosclerosis; 2) structural vascular changes, particularly in the small arterioles; and 3) tubulointerstitial disease. Glomerular damage, e.g., mesangial expansion and basement membrane thickening, is the most characteristic feature of diabetic nephropathy and most often takes the form of diffuse scarring of entire glomeruli. The nodular Kimmelstiel-Wilson glomerularsclerosis, which is considered to be characteristic of diabetic nephropathy, only occurs in a few patients. The tubulointerstitial changes interfere with potassium ion and hydrogen ion secretion and may be at least partly responsible for the hyperkalemia and metabolic acidosis that accompany diabetic renal disease.

NATURAL HISTORY

Shortly after diabetes is diagnosed, the glomerular filtration rate (GFR) and renal blood flow are characteristically elevated, and there is typically a corresponding increase in kidney weight and size. The increased GFR is related to the degree of hyperglycemia, and the GFR is reduced by improved glycemic control. The serum creatinine and urea nitrogen concentrations are slightly reduced because of the renal hyperfiltration. Although a slight increase in urine protein is common when a patient initially presents in diabetic ketoacidosis, once glycemia is well regulated by insulin therapy, proteinuria disappears and remains absent for many yr.

Early in the course of diabetes, the renal histology is normal despite renal hypertrophy. However, within 2–3 yr, many kidneys demonstrate some histological evidence of mesangial expansion and basement membrane thickening. Despite these histologic changes, GFR and renal blood flow may remain elevated, and proteinuria is not detectable. There ensues a long "silent" period (~15 yr) during which there is no laboratory evidence of renal dysfunction. Nonetheless, renal biopsies performed during this period may demonstrate a progressive and widespread increase in the characteristic lesions of diabetic nephropathy. Microalbuminuria (described below) may be present.

Development of Proteinuria

Although the first laboratory evidence of overt diabetic nephropathy is a dipstick-positive urine test (indicating total albuminuria >300 mg in a 24-h period), abnormalities can sometimes be detected even earlier. Because albumin excretion does not exceed 20 mg/day in healthy individuals, there is a wide, subclinical range (20–300 mg/day) of increased urinary albumin excretion rates that go undetected in routine urine testing. The development of more sensitive techniques has permitted the detection of these lower, yet abnormally elevated, albumin excretion rates, referred to as microalbuminuria. Microalbuminuria results vary widely from day to day, and abnormal results should be confirmed by repeat testing.

Patients with diabetes and microalbuminuria are at a higher risk for developing renal insufficiency and may benefit from more intensive follow-up and therapy. However, several factors can induce microalbuminuria, including poor diabetes control, stress, infection, and exercise. These must be excluded before drawing inferences from the presence of microalbuminuria. The presence of even microscopic hematuria is sufficient to invalidate tests for microalbuminuria. Therefore, measurements should not be made during menses or in the presence of urinary tract infection.

Long-Term Prognosis

When routinely detectable proteinuria has developed (>500 mg/day), the long-term prognosis is guarded without institution of a treatment program. Although the GFR may still be elevated at the onset of proteinuria, it usually declines by ~50% within 3 yr, and the serum creatinine and urea nitrogen concentrations become frankly elevated (>2.0 and >30 mg/dl, respectively). Within a mean of 2 yr after the serum creatinine becomes elevated (>2.0 mg/dl), 50% of the individuals will progress to end-stage renal failure. The mean duration of type I diabetes when end-stage renal disease develops is 23 yr. With end-stage renal disease, the uremic symptoms, e.g., drowsiness, lethargy, and nausea, appear and become progressively more pronounced. Most patients receive treatment before reaching this stage, and cardiovascular disease is now the most common cause of death in patients with nephropathy.

Traditionally, it has been considered unusual to observe diabetic nephropathy in the absence of retinopathy, neuropathy, and hypertension. However, the correlation is especially close only in advanced renal disease. As kidney failure progresses, the incidence and severity of all three disorders increases markedly, generally in parallel with renal status.

PATHOGENESIS

Considerable evidence suggests that diabetic nephropathy is related primarily to the metabolic changes induced by the diabetic state. First, renal changes are absent initially in people biopsied around the time of onset of diabetes. Second, typical changes of diabetic nephropathy occur in all types of diabetes. Third, diabetic nephropathy appears in various animal models regardless of whether the diabetes is induced or spontaneous and the damage occurs in both original and transplanted kidneys. Fourth, in these diabetic animals, intensive insulin therapy or islet cell transplantation completely prevents renal histopathologic changes and may reverse early histopathologic abnormalities. Last, improved glucose control can substantially delay the initial appearance of persistent microalbuminunia and clinical grade albuminunia in type I diabetes.

Possible Mechanisms of Damage

The mechanisms by which diabetes damages the kidney remain unknown. It has not been established whether elevated glucose per se or some metabolic event that occurs as a consequence of hyperglycemia is the trigger.

A genetic propensity to diabetic nephropathy may also contribute to its development. Thus, it is possible that metabolic disturbances initiate the processes responsible for diabetic nephropathy but that these processes operate on a genetic background that predisposes to diabetic glomerulosclerosis. Some studies suggest the genetic predisposition relates to an increased familial incidence of essential hypertension.

One explanation for renal damage may involve the typical increases in GFR and renal blood flow that occur early in the course of diabetes. In animals, these alterations in renal hemodynamics are associated with increased intraglomerular pressures. Although it has not been possible to measure intraglomerular pressure in humans, it has been suggested that glomerular hypertension, regardless of what derangements or predispositions lead up to it, is the ultimate mediator of kidney damage in diabetic nephropathy. Measures aimed at reversing the resulting hemodynamic changes have proved useful in slowing the progression of renal disease in human diabetes.

MANAGEMENT

Beginning at diagnosis of diabetes, renal status of all patients with diabetes should be monitored as outlined in Table 6.2. Hypertension should be aggressively treated.

Currently, the management of diabetic nephropathy is largely preventive and supportive. It consists of minimizing factors that are known to accelerate the natural progression of renal disease or that may otherwise jeopardize the kidney and of appropriately responding to changing insulin needs (Tables 6.3 and 6.4). If end-stage renal failure ensues, two options are available: dialysis and kidney transplantation.

HYPERTENSION

In type I diabetes, hypertension typically is secondary to the onset of renal disease. Long-term survivors of diabetes without nephropathy rarely have hypertension. Hypertension is also the single most important factor shown to accelerate the progression of established diabetic nephropathy and contributes to other causes of diabetes-related morbidity and mortality, e.g., retinopathy and heart disease. Aggressive treatment of hypertension is the only therapeutic intervention definitively shown to slow the progression of established renal disease. Therefore, it is paramount that the patient with diabetes have blood pressure normalized (120–130/80 mmHg) to the extent possible without compromising cardiac, cerebral, or other organ-system functions.

Antihypertensive Therapy

The diagnosis of hypertension should be based on multiple blood pressure determinations before beginning treatment. Orthostatic hypotension is frequent in patients with diabetic nephropathy; therefore, both supine and standing blood pressure should be measured. Ambulatory blood pressure monitoring is used in some centers to monitor patients during treatment.

Angiotensin-Converting–Enzyme (ACE) Inhibitors

Recent studies have shown that ACE inhibitors are effective in reducing proteinuria and slowing progression of nephropathy. These drugs may even be effective in patients with microalbuminuria with or without hypertension. ACE inhibitors appear to be the logical first-choice class of drugs for type I diabetic patients with overt nephropathy. However, not all drugs in this class have been prospectively studied for the treatment of nephropathy. Results with captopril in patients with overt nephropathy have conclusively shown a beneficial effect on preserving kidney function. The major serious side effect of ACE inhibitors is hyperkalemia, which is of particular concern in patients with more advanced nephropathy, because they may have the syndrome of hyporeninemic hypoaldosteronism. In the presence of low renin, circulating aldosterone

---

Table 6.2. Monitoring Renal Function

■ *In the first 5 yr of diabetes*, a routine urinalysis with a check for proteinuria should be obtained annually. Serum creatinine and urea nitrogen concentrations should be measured at least once a year if proteinuria is present.

■ *Beyond 5 yr or in the postpubertal patient*, in addition to the above tests, yearly tests for microalbuminuria should be conducted, and if positive, serum creatinine or urea nitrogen concentrations should be measured and glomerular filtration assessed.

■ *Once microalbuminuria (>30 but ≤300 mg/day), overt proteinuria, or elevated serum creatinine or urea nitrogen is detected*, renal function should be monitored at least 2–3 times a year. Consultation with a nephrologist may be helpful to plot a long-term therapeutic strategy and to discuss the possibility and implications of renal failure with the patient if the primary physician or endocrinologist is not expert in the care of patients with nephropathy.

levels are decreased, and the renal tubular secretion of potassium is impaired. Any drug that further impairs aldosterone secretion or action may lead to clinically significant hyperkalemia.

Some patients may experience a precipitous decline in renal function when initiating therapy with ACE inhibitors. Because this appears to be more common in patients with impaired renal function or renovascular hypertension, the physician should determine serum creatinine and potassium levels ~1 wk after therapy begins. An excessive increase in either level warrants discontinuation of the drug.

Diuretics

Because hypertension in the patient with diabetic nephropathy is largely volume sensitive, therapy with a low-sodium diet and a diuretic when edema is present may be effective. Because many hypertensive individuals with diabetes have some degree of renal insufficiency, a loop diuretic is usually necessary. Thiazide diuretics do not promote diuresis once the serum creatinine level has risen to levels >2.0 mg/dl. When used, the dose of thiazide diuretics is lower than that used customarily. Hydrochlorothiazide 12.5 or 25 mg daily is as effective and better tolerated than larger doses. Also, use of diuretics that inhibit potassium secretion (e.g., spironolactone, triamterene) is not recommended for patients with diabetes because of concern for inducing hyperkalemia.

β-Adrenergic–Blocking Agents

β-Adrenergic–blocking agents have also proved successful in treating the hypertensive patient with diabetes. However, this class of drugs inhibits hepatic glucose production, which may lead to hypoglycemia, and they may mask many of the warning symptoms of hypoglycemia (although sweating is not affected). β-Blocking agents also predispose the development of hyperkalemia by inhibiting renin synthesis and impairing potassium uptake by extra renal tissues. Specific β_1-antagonists should be used in patients with diabetes because they are less likely to cause hypoglycemia and hyperkalemia.

Calcium Antagonists

Some studies have shown that calcium antagonists reduce microalbuminuria and proteinuria; however, this effect is variable, and the long-term renal-protective effects are unknown. This class of drugs is relatively free of harmful side effects and does not cause significant alterations in glucose or lipid metabolism. Because of the high incidence of side effects, reserpine and guanethidine should be used with extreme caution in individuals with diabetes.

Table 6.4. Other Threats to Diabetic Kidneys

Several conditions can endanger the kidneys of individuals with diabetes, regardless of whether renal insufficiency has come into play. Among them are the following:

Urinary tract infection. Older individuals with diabetes generally have an increased incidence of urinary tract infection. Therefore, for these patients, it is important that a urinalysis be performed at each clinic visit. If leukocytes or bacteriuria are detected, a urine culture should be obtained. Positive cultures should be treated with an appropriate bactericidal antibiotic.

Neurogenic bladder. The development of a neurogenic bladder is common in patients with diabetes, especially if other evidence of autonomic neuropathy is present, and may predispose to infection. Symptoms (frequent voiding, nocturia, incontinence, recurrent urinary tract infections) may be minimal or may mimic those of prostatic hypertrophy. Once suspected, the diagnosis is easily established if a cystometrogram demonstrates a large atonic bladder with low-pressure recordings.

If the presence of a neurogenic bladder is confirmed, the patient should receive instruction in Credé's manual voiding maneuver, which should be performed every 6–8 h. Often this will be sufficient to prevent postvoid residual and will decompress the upper urinary tract. If not, parasympathetic agents such as bethanechol chloride may be tried. In some people with diabetes, α-adrenergic–blocking agents such as phenoxybenzamine have proved useful. If pharmacologic therapy proves unsuccessful, intermittent straight catheterization should be performed 2–3 times daily.

Intravenous pyelography and other dye studies. Patients with diabetes are at increased risk for acute renal failure after any radiocontrast (intravenous and retrograde pyelography, arteriography, cholangiography, computed tomography scanning) procedure. With the judicious use of echography, radionuclide studies, and noncontrast computed tomography scanning, radiocontrast studies are rarely necessary.

If contrast media must be used, a minimum amount of dye should be given, and adequate hydration should be ensured before the dye study. An osmotic diuresis with mannitol should be started before and continued for 24 h after infusion of the radiocontrast medium. Serum creatinine concentration should be checked daily for 2–3 days after the contrast study.

OTHER ASPECTS OF TREATMENT

Blood Glucose Control

There is no evidence that tight glycemic control through intensive insulin therapy can reverse or even slow the progression of severely advanced renal disease. The DCCT demonstrated conclusively that intensive insulin therapy reduces the development and progression of early renal disease. An intensive treatment program is an essential component of the treatment of a patient found to have microalbuminuria.

The development of renal insufficiency is associated with insulin resistance, and it is common to observe an increase in insulin requirements. As renal failure worsens, it is common to see a decrease in the daily insulin dose and/or an increase in hypoglycemic episodes. For this reason, self-monitoring of blood glucose and use of the results to adjust the insulin dose are important.

Low-Protein Diet

Over the last several yr, there has been renewed interest in the use of low-protein diets to prevent the progression of chronic renal failure (see NUTRITION page 59). The Modification of Diet in Renal Disease Study of nondiabetic patients with advanced renal failure (creatinine clearance <25 ml/min) showed that a restricted protein intake has a palliative effect on the progression of kidney failure. Recent studies in patients with diabetes have also demonstrated that low-protein diets reduce proteinuria and the rate of decline in renal function.

A low-protein diet must be high in carbohydrate and/or fat; however, the long-term effects of such a diet on atherosclerotic complications and glycemia control are unknown. Similarly, it is not known whether a low-protein diet can maintain a normal nitrogen balance in a diabetic patient with advanced renal insufficiency.

Low-protein diets are difficult for the patient to maintain, and a modest restriction in dietary protein combined with the other treatment measures may be more reasonable.

DIALYSIS AND KIDNEY TRANSPLANTATION

Once end-stage renal failure ensues, prolonging life requires dialysis or a functioning kidney transplant. The pros and cons of these procedures should be discussed with patients and their families well in advance of end-stage renal failure. The prospect of needing such measures should never be a surprise. The ultimate choice among alternatives requires input from the patient, the patient's family, a nephrologist, and the primary-care physician. Absolute indications for dialysis or transplantation include serum creatinine >8 mg/dl or creatinine clearance of ≤10 ml/min as well as urgent uremic symptoms, e.g., seizures, uremic pericarditis, unresponsive hypertension, and muscle deterioration. More subjective criteria include worsening lethargy, nausea or vomiting, and progressive retinopathy and neuropathy. The general trend is to not delay the start of dialysis in patients with diabetes and begin earlier than in patients without diabetes.

Renal Dialysis

Of the various forms of renal dialysis, hemodialysis is the most frequently used in diabetic patients, although various forms of peritoneal dialysis have also been used with success. There are considerable data to suggest that adequate delivery of dialytic therapy is critical for survival. Delivered KT/V of 1.2–1.4 appears to be a minimal goal for diabetic patients. Some patients using intermittent or continuous ambulatory peritoneal dialysis (CAPD) have insulin included with the dialysate. This procedure often improves blood glucose control because peritoneal insulin delivery is more physiologic than subcutaneous delivery. CAPD also affords a motivated patient the greatest mobility, although its long-term efficacy in comparison with other dialysis techniques is still under study. Treatment of anemia with erythropoietin has substantially improved the general well-being of patients on dialysis.

Kidney Transplantation

When the success rate of kidney transplantation in patients with diabetes approached the excellent success rate achieved in patients without diabetes, this procedure became the treatment of choice in young patients with diabetic end-stage renal disease. Kidneys donated by first-degree relatives continue to be preferable, although increasing experience with immunosuppressive agents has helped lower the incidence of rejection with tissue-matched cadaver-donated kidneys.

The decision of whether to opt for a transplant is still not one to be taken lightly, and a patient must be well briefed on the enhances of failure, as well as the probability (for younger patients) that the new kidney will undergo the same changes that caused the original kidney to fail. This risk means that the post-transplantation patient should be considered for initiation of an intensive insulin-treatment program. The options available in the event of end-stage renal failure offer greater possibilities than were available even 5 yr ago for salvaging quality of life and increasing longevity.

Kidney transplantation can often be successfully combined with pancreas transplantation. Combination transplantation increases short-term morbidity, but properly selected patients may have better long-term rehabilitation.

CONCLUSION

End-stage renal disease is a major cause of morbidity and mortality in patients with type I diabetes of >15 yr duration. Vigilant monitoring of evolving proteinuria and in particular its early detection with microalbuminuria testing, striving for excellent glycemic control within patient-acceptable goals, aggressive therapy of hypertension, and anticipating the need for dialysis or transplantation form the cornerstones of management. The primary-care provider is pivotal in integrating available resources, including referral to a nephrologist.

BIBLIOGRAPHY

American Diabetes Association consensus statement: Treatment of hypertension in diabetes. *Diabetes Care* 16:1364–401, 1993

Bojestig M, Arnqvist HJ, Hermansson G, et al.: Declining incidence of nephropathy in insulin-dependent diabetes mellitus. *N Engl J Med* 330:15–18, 1994

Cohen D, Dodds R, Viberti G: Effect of protein restriction in insulin dependent diabetics at risk of nephropathy. *Br Med J* 294:795–98, 1987

DCCT Research Group: The effect of intensive treatment of diabetes on the development and progression of long-term complications in insulin-dependent diabetes mellitus. *N Engl J Med* 329:977–86, 1993

Kasiske BL, Kalikl RSN, Ma JZ, et al.: Effect of antihypertensive therapy on the kidney in patients with diabetes: a meta-regression analysis. *Ann Intern Med* 118:129–38, 1993

Klahr S, Levey AS, Bejck GJ, Caggiula AW, Hunsicker L, Kusek JW, Striker G, The Modification of Diet and Renal Disease Study Group: The effects of dietary protein restriction and blood pressure control on the progression of chronic renal disease. *N Engl J Med* 330:877–84, 1994

Kopple JD, Hakim RM, Held PJ, Keane WF, King K, Lazarus JM, Parker TF, Teehan BP: National Kidney Foundation position paper: Recommendations for reducing the high morbidity and mortality of U.S. maintenance hemodialysis patients. *Am J Kidney Dis*. In press

Lewis JL, Hunsicker LG, Bain RP: The effect of angiotensin-converting-enzyme inhibition on diabetic nephropathy. *N Engl J Med* 329:1456–62, 1993

Mogensen CE, Christensen CK: Predicating diabetic nephropathy in insulin-dependent patients. *N Engl J Med* 311:89–93, 1984

Viberti GC, Wiseman MJ: The kidney in diabetes: significance of the early abnormalities. *Clin Endocrinol Metab* 15:753–82, 1986

The Working Group on Hypertension in Diabetes: Statement on hypertension in diabetes mellitus. *Arch Intern Med* 147:830–42, 1987

Zatz R, Brenner BM: Pathogenesis of diabetic microangiopathy: the hemodynamic view. *Am J Med* 80:443–53, 1986

Neuropathy

INTRODUCTION

Peripheral neuropathy is one of the most common and troubling chronic complications of diabetes. Virtually all regions of the body can be affected by diabetic neuropathy, which can produce significant impairments alone and in concert with other conditions. Most notably, neuropathic loss of sensation in the foot regularly conspires with infection and/or vascular insufficiency (more common in people with diabetes) to make diabetes the most frequent source of nontraumatic lower-limb amputations in the United States.

OVERVIEW OF NEUROPATHIES

The frequency of diabetic neuropathy parallels duration and severity of hyperglycemia in both type I and II diabetes. In patients with type I diabetes, it rarely occurs within the first 5 yr after diagnosis. The exception is a patient with prolonged, very poor control early in the course of diabetes. These patients often develop painful neuropathy. Sometimes the symptoms become manifest only after the initiation of insulin therapy. Neuropathy in diabetes can also be caused by pancreatectomy, nonalcoholic pancreatitis, and hemochromatosis, as well as independently in conditions more commonly associated with type I diabetes, e.g., hypothyroidism and pernicious anemia.

Histological Findings

Histologically, there is loss of both large and small myelinated nerve fibers, accompanied by varying degrees of paranodal and segmental demyelination, connective tissue proliferation, and thickening and reduplication of capillary basement membranes with capillary closure. Researchers are investigating several potential pathways by which hyperglycemia (perhaps aided by other metabolic derangements of diabetes) may cause such changes. The polyol pathway, protein glycation, and altered intracellular oxidation-reduction potential are prominent among the mechanisms being studied.

Treatment of Neuropathies

There is no known direct treatment for neuropathy. The DCCT demonstrated that intensive treatment programs reduce by 60% the development and progression of early neuropathy. Dietary supplements of *myo*-inositol have been suggested based on animal studies, but fragmentary clinical experience has not been encouraging. Aldose reductase inhibitors, which block the accumulation of sorbitol and loss of *myo*-inositol from diabetic nerve and improve nerve conduction in diabetic animals and patients, are undergoing clinical trials in symptomatic neuropathy; however, the trials to date have shown only modest effectiveness in more advanced forms of neuropathy. Earlier long-term interventions are being studied with various agents.

Clinical Syndrome

Diabetic neuropathy is classified into a set of discrete clinical syndromes, each with a characteristic presentation and clinical course (Table 6.5). Because the syndromes overlap clinically and frequently occur simultaneously, rigid classification of individual cases is often difficult. Identical neurological syndromes occur in other diseases and other conditions. For example, alcoholic neuropathy and inflammatory neuropathies can mimic peripheral diabetic neuropathy. Diabetic neuropathy is a diagnosis of exclusion (Table 6.6).

DISTAL SYMMETRIC SENSORIMOTOR POLYNEUROPATHY

Distal symmetric polyneuropathy is the most common form of diabetic neuropathy. Sensory signs and symptoms generally predominate over motor involvement and vary depending on the classes of nerve fibers. Loss of large fibers produces diminished proprioception and light touch, resulting in ataxic gait, unsteadiness, and weakness of intrinsic muscles in the hands and feet. Involvement of small fibers causes diminished pain and temperature sensation, resulting in unrecognized trauma (especially to the feet), accidental burning of the hands, etc.

Typical neuropathic paresthesia (spontaneous uncomfortable sensations) or dysesthesia (contact paresthesia) may accompany both large- and small-fiber involvement. Sensory deficits first appear in the most distal portions of the extremities and spread proximally with disease progression in a "stocking-glove" distribution. In the most advanced cases, vertical bands of sensory deficit develop on the chest or abdomen when the tips of the shorter truncal nerves become involved (Figure 6.9).

Occasionally, patients complain of exquisite hypersensitivity to light touch, superficial burning or stabbing pain, or bone-deep aching or tearing pain, usually most troublesome at night. Sometimes, neuropathic pain may become the overriding and disabling feature, especially in small-fiber neuropathy. Both neuropathic pain and paresthesia are thought to reflect spontaneous depolarization of newly regenerating nerve fibers.

Asymptomatic Neuropathy

Many patients with distal symmetrical polyneuropathy remain free of troubling, subjective symptoms. In these cases, it may take careful questioning to learn of

---

Table 6.5. Syndromes of Diabetic Neuropathy

Diffuse neuropathies (common, insidious onset, usually progressive)
- Distal symmetrical sensorimotor polyneuropathy
- Autonomic neuropathy

Focal neuropathies (sudden onset, usually improve over time)
- Cranial neuropathy
- Radiculopathy
- Plexopathy
- Mononeuropathy/mononeuropathy multiplex
  - Other mononeuropathies

---

a patient's subtle feelings of numbness or cold or "dead" feet. Diminished or absent deep-tendon reflexes, especially the Achilles-tendon reflex, is often an early indication of otherwise asymptomatic neuropathy. However, in the absence of pain or paresthesia, diabetic neuropathy may go unrecognized unless the physician routinely tests foot sensation during office visits.

LATE COMPLICATIONS OF POLYNEUROPATHY

Patients with chronic, unrecognized neuropathy may present with late complications, e.g., foot ulceration, foreign

---

Table 6.6. Common Conditions Resembling Various Forms of Diabetic Neuropathy

Distal symmetrical neuropathy
- Inflammatory neuropathies (vasculitic, i.e., systemic lupus erythematosis, polyarteritis, and other connective tissue diseases; sarcoidosis; leprosy)
- Metabolic neuropathies (hypothyroidism, uremic; nutritional; acute intermittent porphyric)
- Toxic neuropathies (alcohol; drugs; heavy metals, e.g., lead, mercury, and arsenic; industrial hydrocarbons)
- Other neuropathies (paraneoplastic; dysproteinemic, amyloid, hereditary)

Autonomic neuropathy
- Idiopathic orthostatic hypotension
- Shy-Drager syndrome (progressive autonomic failure)

Cranial neuropathy
- Carotid aneurysm
- Intracranial mass
- Elevated intracranial pressure

Radiculopathy
- Spinal cord/root compression
- Transverse myelitis
- Coagulopathies
- Shingles

Plexopathy
- Mass lesions
- Coagulopathies
- Cauda equina lesions (femoral neuropathy)

Mononeuropathy/mononeuropathy multiplex
- Compression neuropathies
- Inflammatory (vasculitic) neuropathies
- Hypothyroidism, acromegaly

Figure 6.9. Distribution of Sensory Loss in Patient With Severe Chronic Diabetic Sensory Polyneuropathy

Loss is maximal distally in limbs but also affects anterior trunk and vertex of head. *Hatched lines*, pinprick impaired; *crosshatched lines*, pinprick absent; *stippled lines*, hyperesthesia. *From* Sabin TD, Geschwind M, Waxman SG: Patterns of clinical deficits in peripheral nerve disease. In *Physiology and Pathophysiology of Axons*. New York, Raven, 1987, p. 431–38

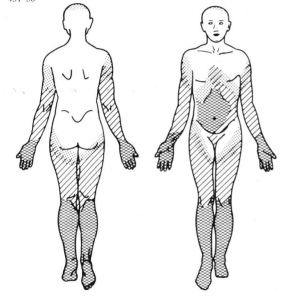

objects embedded in the foot, unrecognized trauma to the extremities, or neuroarthropathy (Charcot's joints). All of these conditions are avoidable with proper early diagnosis of neuropathy and institution of appropriate foot care.

Foot Ulcerations and Infections

Acute foot ulcerations and resulting infections can occur when an individual cannot feel the pain due to poorly fitting shoes (a source of penetrating abrasions), a retained foreign body, or accidental trauma (often unintentionally self-inflicted during nail trimming) because of neuropathy. Plantar ulcers, which form at the calloused sites of maximal walking pressure, can result from a combination of motor, cutaneous sensory, and proprioceptive deficits.

Patients with long-standing diabetes and neuropathy are also predisposed to vascular ulcers due to macrovascular and microvascular insufficiency and ischemic gangrene.

In a typical sequence of events, imbalance of extensor and flexor muscles in the feet, resulting from impaired proprioception and atrophy of intrinsic extensor muscles, leads to tendon shortening and chronic toe flexion (claw-toe or hammer-toe deformity). This, in turn, shifts weight bearing from the padded ball of the foot to the unprotected metatarsal heads. With pain insensitivity, trauma to the overlying skin goes undetected, producing thick callouses that further concentrate weight bearing over the bony prominences. Splitting and fissuring of the thick callus or underlying pressure necrosis initiates ulcer formation, further aggravated by infection and vascular insufficiency.

Neuroarthropathy

Neuroarthropathy refers to the joint erosions, unrecognized fractures, demineralization, and devitalization of bones in the foot resulting from ignoring the minor injuries that occur during routine daily weight-bearing activities. Neuropathy impairs normal protective proprioceptive and nociceptive functions, which should lead the patient to recognize the injury and protect the foot. The foot may be swollen and red, but it is not painful. The problem may be misdiagnosed as cellulitis despite a normal leukocyte count and differential and the absence of fever. The patient may report relatively painless trauma, and initial radiographic examination may be unrevealing, whereas follow-up X rays several days or weeks later may reveal clear traumatic changes. In more advanced cases, devitalization of bone may mimic osteomyelitis, and in the most advanced stages, the foot may look like a "bag of bones."

MANAGEMENT OF DISTAL SYMMETRIC POLYNEUROPATHY AND COMPLICATIONS

Treatment for diabetic distal symmetric polyneuropathy is symptomatic, palliative, and supportive, with primary emphasis on preventing the late complications. In most cases, the primary neuropathic symptoms consist of mild intermittent pain or paresthesia. Even severely painful symptoms generally remit spontaneously within a few months in most but not all patients.

Management of Pain

Persistent and severely painful neuropathy has been treated with various drugs, including standard analgesics and drugs normally used to treat pain in other conditions. Narcotics should be avoided except in the most extreme cases. Subantidepressive doses of amitriptyline or other antidepressants are helpful in some but not all patients and should be given a short therapeutic trial. Although not substantiated by controlled clinical trials, the anticonvulsant carbamazepine has been used based on its membrane-stabilizing properties. The antiarrhythmic drug mexilitene may have similar effectiveness. Topical capsaicin applied frequently to the hypersensitive areas often decreases pain. Transcutaneous electrical nerve stimulation has also been used for refractory painful neuropathy. Other physical therapy measures such as contrast baths and stretching exercises provide ancillary help.

Because early diagnosis of asymptomatic neuropathy is essential for preventing the late complications, every routine physician visit should include a thorough examination of the feet if the patient has preexisting risk factors or any foot symptoms. A list of neurologic and related symptoms to watch for is given in Table 6.7.

Callus Formation and Plantar Ulcers

Callus formation over weight-bearing areas indicates the need to consult a podiatrist and/or orthopedist for prescription of corrective footwear to redistribute weight bearing. Plantar ulcers should be managed by eliminating weight bearing either by special walking casts or by bed rest. Local debridement and application of platelet-derived growth factors may speed healing.

Refractory and/or recurrent ulcers may be managed by surgical removal of the involved metatarsal. If there is evidence of impaired macrovascular circulation, vascular studies should be obtained and revascularization attempted when indicated. Neuroarthropathy is managed by reduced ambulation and weight bearing, as well as cushioned footwear.

Treatment of Infection

Infection must be treated aggressively with appropriate consultation from infectious-disease specialists. Antibiotics effective against anaerobic organisms should be included in the treatment regimen. Deep-wound cultures are necessary to direct antibiotic therapy properly. Vascular bypass surgery or percutaneous angioplasty should be considered if arterial insufficiency is a major contributing factor. Localized osteomyelitis may require a limited amputation.

AUTONOMIC NEUROPATHY

Neuropathy can affect virtually any autonomic function in patients with diabetes. Although autonomic neuropathy produces diffuse subclinical dysfunction, autonomic symptoms are usually confined to one or two organ systems, producing the discrete autonomic syndromes listed in Table 6.8.

Cardiovascular Autonomic Neuropathy

The earliest clinical signs of cardiovascular autonomic neuropathy are absence of the normal sleep bradycardia and diminished variation of the pulse rate with inspiration-expiration or Valsalva (reduced sinus tachycardia), both due to early vagal involvement.

Later, sympathetic denervation interferes with normal cardiovascular reflexes thereby diminishing exercise tolerance, possibly hypersensitizing the heart to circulating catecholamines, tachyarrhythmias, and sudden death. It also predisposes to painless myocardial infarction.

Table 6.7. Warning Symptoms and Signs of Diabetic Foot Problems

	SYMPTOMS	SIGNS
Vascular	■ Cold feet ■ Intermittent claudication involving calf or foot ■ Pain at rest, especially nocturnal, relieved by dependency	■ Absent pedal, popliteal, or femoral pulses ■ Femoral bruits ■ Dependent rubor, plantar pallor on elevation ■ Prolonged capillary filling time (>3–4 s) ■ Decreased skin temperature
Neurologic	■ Sensory: burning, tingling, or crawling sensations; pain and hypersensitivity; complaints of cold or "dead" feet ■ Motor: weakness (drop foot) ■ Autonomic: diminished sweating	■ Sensory: deficits (vibratory and proprio perceptive, then pain and temperature perception), hyperesthesia ■ Motor: diminished to absent deep-tendon reflexes (Achilles then patellar), weakness ■ Autonomic: diminished to absent sweating
Musculoskeletal	■ Gradual change in foot shape ■ Sudden painless change in foot shape, with swelling, without history of trauma	■ Cavus feet with claw toes ■ Drop foot ■ "Rocker-bottom" foot (Charcot's joint) ■ Neuropathic arthropathy
Dermatologic	■ Exquisitely painful or painless wounds ■ Slow-healing or nonhealing wounds, necrosis ■ Skin color changes (cyanosis, redness) ■ Chronic scaling, itching, or dry feet ■ Recurrent infections (e.g, paronychia, athlete's foot)	Skin ■ Abnormal dryness ■ Chronic tinea infections ■ Keratotic lesions with or without hemorrhage (plantar or digital) ■ Trophic ulcer Hair ■ Diminished to absent Nails ■ Trophic changes ■ Onychomycosis ■ Subungual ulceration or abcess ■ Ingrown nails with paronychia

From Scardina RJ: Diabetic foot problems: assessment and prevention. *Clin Diabetes* 1:1–7, 1983

Orthostatic Hypotension

Orthostatic hypotension is managed by correcting hypovolemia with fluid replacement and improved diabetes control, elastic stockings, increased salt intake, mineralocorticoids, or vasoconstrictors.

Gastrointestinal Autonomic Neuropathy

Nonspecific gastrointestinal symptoms in diabetic patients often reflect diffuse but subtle gastrointestinal autonomic dysfunction. Esophageal dysmotility can cause dysphagia, retrosternal discomfort, and heartburn.

Delayed gastric emptying (gastroparesis) causes anorexia, nausea, vomiting, early satiety, and postprandial bloating and fullness. Delayed nutrient absorption can greatly complicate glycemic control, producing otherwise unexplained swings between severe hyperglycemia and hypoglycemia.

Diagnosis

Diagnosis of upper gastrointestinal symptoms requires liquid- and solid-phase radionuclide gastric-emptying studies. Diagnostic studies of lower gastrointestinal problems are necessary to define the multiple contributing factors that stem from widespread intestinal autonomic dysfunction to determine appropriate treatment.

Treatment

Management of esophageal dysmotility and delayed gastric emptying includes frequent small and/or primarily liquid feedings. High-fiber diets should be avoided, because they delay gastric emptying and may form bezoars. Dopamine antagonists such as metoclopramide or cisipride or parasympathetic agonists may be helpful. A therapeutic trial of broad-spectrum antibiotics may also be helpful, whereas evidence of bile salt malabsorption would argue in favor of bile salt–sequestering agents, both of which are effective in properly selected patients. Hypermotility is managed with diphenoxylate hydrochloride.

Constipation/Diarrhea

Diabetic constipation is the most frequent gastrointestinal complaint, occurring in 60% of patients with diabetes. Stool softeners and laxatives or cathartics used judiciously are usually effective, although dopamine antagonists are occasionally indicated.

Diabetic diarrhea is classically painless, nocturnal, associated with fecal incontinence, and alternates with periods of constipation. Fecal incontinence, which is also usually nocturnal, reflects impaired sensation of rectal distention, and in one small series of patients, it was effectively managed with biofeedback techniques.

Sexual Dysfunction

Erectile Impotence

Erectile impotence in diabetic men may be psychogenic, endocrine, vascular, drug or stress related, or neuropathic. Normal erections on awakening or impotence only with a certain partner suggests a psychogenic cause. A band-type turgidity gauge or nocturnal penile tumescence monitoring at a sleep research facility can help clarify ambiguous situations.

Table 6.8. Syndromes of Autonomic Neuropathy

Cardiovascular autonomic neuropathy
- Resting sinus tachycardia without sinus arrhythmia (fixed heart rate)
- Exercise intolerance
- Painless myocardial infarction
- Orthostatic hypotension
- Sudden death

Gastrointestinal autonomic neuropathy
- Esophageal dysfunction
- Autonomic gastropathy and delayed gastric emptying
- Diabetic diarrhea
- Constipation
- Fecal incontinence
- Gallbladder atony

Genitourinary autonomic neuropathy
- Erectile impotence
- Retrograde ejaculation with infertility
- Bladder dysfunction

Hypoglycemia unawareness

Sudomotor neuropathy
- Facial sweating
- Heat intolerance
- "Gustatory" sweating

Sex steroid imbalances, hypogonadotrophism, and hyperprolactinemia should be excluded by appropriate endocrine studies. Proximal vascular insufficiency is usually evident on examination of the femoral pulses, although localized obstruction of the penile artery has been reported and can be excluded only by measurement of the brachial-penile blood pressure ratio with Doppler-flow studies. Proximal or localized vascular obstruction has been managed surgically, but the success rate is low.

Drugs known to produce impotence include various antihypertensives, anticholinergics, antipsychotics, antidepressants, narcotics, barbiturates, alcohol, and amphetamines. Neuropathic impotence is generally but not always accompanied by other manifestations of diabetic neuropathy.

Management

Drug-induced impotence is managed by altering the treatment regimen when possible. Neuropathic impotence is managed by appropriate counseling and penile prostheses when indicated.

A nonsurgical technique involving a vacuum device and elastic constriction of the penis is successful in men with diabetes, although its long-term safety is still being assessed. Injection of papaverine or other vasoactive drugs directly into the corpus cavernosum can stimulate erection in neuropathic impotence and is another successful, well-accepted treatment method.

Retrograde Ejaculation
Retrograde ejaculation, which may or may not occur in conjunction with impotence, reflects loss of the coordinated closure of the internal and relaxation of the external vesicle sphincter during ejaculation. Presentation is usually infertility, and diagnosis is confirmed by documenting ejaculate azoospermia and the presence of motile sperm in postcoital urine. Such sperm have been successfully used for artificial insemination.

Other Autonomic Syndromes

Diabetic Cystopathy
Cystopathy initially diminishes sensation of bladder fullness, reducing urinary frequency. Later, efferent involvement produces incomplete urination, poor stream, dribbling, and overflow incontinence, and it predisposes to urinary tract infections.

Conservative management involves scheduled voluntary urination with or without Credé's maneuver. Cholinergic-stimulating drugs, sphincter relaxants, periodic catheterization, and bladder-neck resection of the internal sphincter may be used in more advanced cases.

Hypoglycemia Unawareness
Hypoglycemia unawareness may be related to autonomic neuropathy, which can blunt the usual adrenergic response to hypoglycemia. This is generally conceded to predispose to severe hypoglycemia and may be a contraindication to intensive insulin treatment.

Autonomic Sudomotor Dysfunction
Autonomic sudomotor dysfunction produces an asymptomatic anhidrosis of the extremities and compensatory central hyperhidrosis. It diminishes thermoregulatory reserve and predisposes to heat stroke and hyperthermia. Management is confined to avoidance of heat stress.

FOCAL NEUROPATHIES

Neural deficits corresponding to the distribution of single or multiple peripheral nerves (mononeuropathy and mononeuropathy multiplex), cranial nerves, areas of the brachial or lumbosacral plexuses (plexopathy), or the nerve roots (radiculopathy) are of sudden onset and generally but not always self-limiting in patients with diabetes.

The third cranial nerve may be affected, presenting with unilateral pain, diplopia, and ptosis but with pupillary sparing. Differential diagnosis includes an aneurysm of the internal carotid artery and myasthenia gravis. Spontaneous remission usually occurs within a few months.

Radiculopathy
Radiculopathy presents as bandlike thoracic or abdominal pain, often misdiagnosed as an acute intrathoracic or intra-abdominal emergency.

Femoral Neuropathy
Femoral neuropathy in patients with diabetes often involves motor and sensory deficits at the level of the sacral plexus as well as the femoral nerve, with the relative excess of motor versus sensory involvement differentiating diabetic femoral neuropathy from that seen in other conditions. When bilateral, this is sometimes termed *amyotrophy*. Management of focal neuropathies includes exclusion of other causes, e.g., nerve entrapment or compression and symptomatic palliation pending spontaneous resolution, which occurs generally but not always over periods of months to yr.

CONCLUSION

Diabetic neuropathy is an extremely common complication of diabetes that becomes more prevalent with increasing duration and severity of hyperglycemia. Its manifestations include diffuse and focal painful and painless neurological deficits in the peripheral nervous system and widespread autonomic dysfunction. Prompt and proper diagnosis is essential to effective management and avoidance of serious secondary musculoskeletal and visceral complications.

BIBLIOGRAPHY

DCCT Research Group: The effect of intensive treatment of diabetes on the development and progression of long-term complications in insulin-dependent diabetes mellitus. *N Engl J Med* 329:977–86, 1993

Dyck PJ, Thomas PK, Asbury AK, Winegrad AI, Porte D, (Eds.): *Diabetic Neuropathy*. Philadelphia, PA, Saunders, 1987

Elements RS: Diabetic neuropathy: diagnosis and treatment. *Clin Diabetes* 2:73–92, 1984

Greene DA, Lattimer SA, Sima AAF: Sorbitol phosphoinositides and Na-K-ATPase in pathogenesis of diabetic complications. *N Engl J Med* 316:599–606, 1987

Hilsted J, Richter E, Madsbad S: Metabolic and cardiovascular responses to epinephrine in diabetic autonomic neuropathy. *N Engl J Med* 317:421–26, 1987

Pfeifer MA, Ross DR, Schrage JP, Gelber DA, Schumer MP, Crain GM, Markwell SJ, Jung S: A highly successful and novel model for treatment of chronic painful diabetic peripheral neuropathy. *Diabetes Care* 16: 1103–15, 1993

Von der Ohe M, Camilleri MD, Zimmerman BR: Management of diabetic enteropathy. *Endocrinologist* 6:400–408, 1993

Macrovascular Disease

INTRODUCTION

Coronary heart disease, peripheral vascular disease, and cerebrovascular disease are more common, tend to occur at an earlier age, and are more extensive and severe in people with diabetes. Diabetes itself is a risk factor for atherosclerotic cardiovascular disease (ASCVD). Other risk factors include hypertension, which is more prevalent in people with type I diabetes than in the general population; cigarette smoking, which is as common among diabetic people as in the general population; and abnormalities of lipid metabolism.

PREVALENCE AND RISK FACTORS

Although cardiovascular deaths are less common in patients with type I diabetes than in generally older type II diabetic patients, mortality rates among type I diabetic individuals are, nonetheless, >11 times greater than among individuals of the same age without diabetes. ASCVD accounts for ~25% of deaths among patients with onset of diabetes before age 20 yr. Heart disease causes 27% and strokes cause 6% of deaths among diabetic patients under age 45 yr. Many of these deaths occur in patients with diabetic nephropathy, and a large percentage of them result from the interaction of diabetes, hypertension, and cigarette smoking.

Diabetes is an independent risk factor for ASCVD, increasing risk two- to threefold. Diabetic women are at special risk. They lose the normal "protection" of female sex, and their cardiovascular disease rates, even before menopause, parallel those of diabetic men.

The prevalence of lipid abnormalities varies significantly depending on the characteristics of the study population such as age, sex, type of diabetes, level of obesity, glycemic control, drugs, and thyroid and renal status. In patients with type I diabetes and good glycemic control, lipid levels are no different from an age- and sex-matched control population. In fact, with excellent control, the lipid profile may show lower total cholesterol and higher high-density lipoprotein (HDL) cholesterol levels than in control subjects. Levels of cholesterol, ratios of total cholesterol to HDL cholesterol, and triglyceride levels are generally higher in type I diabetic patients during periods of poor glycemic control and are powerful risk factors for cardiovascular disease. Diabetic ketoacidosis may be associated with profound, temporary hypertriglyceridemia. When even minimal proteinuria is present, the lipid levels may reveal an atherogenic profile. The most extreme example is with the nephrotic syndrome. Even when the lipid levels are acceptable by conventional measures, glycation of lipoproteins and other lipoprotein compositional abnormalities induced by diabetes may make them more atherogenic.

Hypertension and cigarette smoking are major cardiovascular risk factors. In health surveys of people aged 20–44 yr, 29% of those with diabetes (compared to only 8% of those without diabetes) report having hypertension. Fortunately, the percentage of smokers is decreasing, but young patients with diabetes should frequently be reminded not to begin this habit.

In the DCCT, intensively treated type I diabetic patients with lower HbA_{1c} levels had trends toward lower levels of low-density lipoprotein cholesterol and fewer myocardial infarctions and peripheral vascular events.

ASSESSMENT AND TREATMENT

Because of the high prevalence of risk factors, physicians should consider all patients with type I diabetes to be at risk for developing macrovascular disease. They should systematically assess patients for risk factors for ASCVD (those mentioned above plus a family history of cardiovascular disease or hyperlipidemia), question them about symptoms of ASCVD, and be alert for signs of atherosclerosis. When appropriate, a program for modifying risk factors should be started.

Dyslipidemia

Dyslipidemia in a diabetic patient may result from poor metabolic control; use of certain drugs, e.g., β-blockers or estrogens; obesity; associated conditions such as hypothyroidism; or an independent inborn error of lipid metabolism. Each cause must be considered in assessing diabetic patients for high blood lipid levels.

In 1993, the American Diabetes Association published a consensus statement on the detection and management of lipid disorders in diabetes. It was recommended that adult patients with diabetes should be tested annually for lipid disorders with a fasting serum cholesterol, triglyceride, and HDL cholesterol determination. Children should be tested after the diagnosis of diabetes once reasonable glycemic control is achieved and annually only if abnormalities are identified.

If dyslipidemia is present, the patient should be assessed for factors that aggrevate hyper- or dyslipidemia. Insulin treatment should be intensified because elevated triglyceride and cholesterol levels will return toward normal and HDL cholesterol levels will rise with intensification of insulin therapy in poorly controlled patients. Any drugs that might exacerbate hyperlipidemia, e.g., thiazide diuretics, should be discontinued, and the patient should be evaluated for renal disease and alcohol abuse. Genetic hyperlipidemia, separate from the diabetes, is often the cause of marked hypercholesterolemia, and the treatment should be based on the etiology of the disorder.

The physician should also determine whether the patient is following the current American Diabetes Association guidelines regarding fat intake (see NUTRITION, Table 3.9). Risk categories and recommendations for treatment can be found in Table 6.9.

Hypertension

Blood pressure should be measured in all patients with type I diabetes, including children and adolescents, at each physical examination or at least every 6 mo and hypertension treatment should be initiated to reduce the risk of macrovascular and microvascular dis-

ease. To the extent possible, blood pressure should be maintained at levels <140/90 mmHg in adults or below the 95th percentile for age- and sex-adjusted norms. When prescribing pharmacologic therapy, the clinician should consider the adverse effects of various antihypertensive drugs on hyperglycemia and hypoglycemia, electrolyte balance, renal function, lipid metabolism, ASCVD, and neuropathic symptoms including orthostatic hypotension and impotence.

Cigarette Smoking

Each patient's smoking history should also be determined. Nonsmokers, particularly children and adolescents, should be encouraged not to begin, and smokers should be strongly urged to stop. The physician's advice not to smoke has an impact and represents time well spent. Advice should be reinforced with educational materials, with referral to a smoking-cessation program, and by prohibiting smoking in the physician office.

SYMPTOMS AND SIGNS OF ATHEROSCLEROSIS

The physician should be particularly alert to the symptoms and signs of atherosclerosis in all patients with diabetes.

Cerebrovascular Disease

Symptoms of cerebrovascular disease include intermittent dizziness, transient loss of vision, slurring of speech, and paresthesia or weakness of one arm or leg. Vascular bruits may be heard over the carotid arteries. Noninvasive procedures, including Doppler and carotid ultrasound studies, may help to determine the diagnosis.

Aspirin at a dose of 325 mg daily may prevent a recurrence of symptoms, and use of anticoagulant medications after a transient ischemic attack may help some patients. Angiography may be indicated when surgery is being considered, but the therapeutic value of surgical approaches to cerebrovascular

Table 6.9. Lipid Levels for Adults

RISK FOR ADULT DIABETIC PATIENTS	CHOLESTEROL (mg/dl)	HDL CHOLESTEROL (mg/dl)	LDL CHOLESTEROL (mg/dl)	TRIGLYCERIDES (mg/dl)
Acceptable	<200	—	<130	<200
Borderline	200–239	—	130–159	200–399
High	≥240	≤35	≥160	≥400

HDL, high-density lipoprotein; LDL, low-density lipoprotein.
From American Diabetes Association consensus statement: see Bibliography

disease has not been shown to be superior to standard medical therapy.

Coronary Heart Disease

As in people without type I diabetes, coronary heart disease may be associated with chest pain or congestive heart failure. However, among people with diabetes, ischemia may occur in the absence of chest pain and particularly in the presence of cardiac autonomic neuropathy. Unexplained onset of congestive heart failure and deterioration of glycemic control to the point of diabetic ketoacidosis may indicate silent myocardial ischemia, and myocardial infarction should be considered in the differential diagnosis of these conditions. Noninvasive procedures, including exercise tolerance tests, exercise thallium studies, and gated blood pool scans, may help establish the diagnosis of silent ischemia and/or myocardial perfusion defects. The utility, frequency, and cost-benefit ratios of these studies in older, asymptomatic patients to screen for coronary artery disease has not been determined.

Therapy may be medical or surgical. Medical treatments include aspirin, nitrates, calcium-channel blockers, and cardioselective β-adrenergic blockers. Coronary angiography is necessary if bypass surgery or angioplasty is being considered. Bypass surgery or angioplasty is recommended for left main coronary artery disease and is often indicated for triple-vessel disease, particularly in the presence of left ventricular dysfunction.

Peripheral Vascular Disease

Peripheral vascular disease should be suspected in patients who complain of buttock, calf, or thigh pain that occurs during exercise and is relieved with rest (intermittent claudication) and/or who exhibit decreased pulses in the lower extremities. The diagnosis can be confirmed with noninvasive Doppler studies.

An expert panel of the American Heart Association has recommended regular determination of ankle/brachial index in type I diabetic patients over age 35 yr. Sclerotic vessels can lead to falsely elevated systolic blood pressure and invalid results. Otherwise, a decreased index not only indicates a patient with peripheral vascular disease but is also a strong indicator of possible coronary artery disease.

Treatment with pentoxifylline may improve symptoms. Aspirin and exercise are important adjuvants to treatment. If pain is incapacitating or persists at rest, or if a foot infection results from impaired blood flow through the major leg arteries, angioplasty or surgery to bypass the diseased vessels may be indicated. For more information on foot care, see EDUCATION and NEUROPATHY.

CONCLUSION

Patients with type I diabetes should be aware of their increased risk of ASCVD and advised of the importance of modifying risk factors such as hypertension, hyperlipidemia, and cigarette smoking. Clinicians should systematically assess patients for risk factors for ASCVD and attempt to modify them. They should question patients about symptoms of ASCVD, examine them for signs of ASCVD, and seek the expertise of appropriate specialists when needed.

BIBLIOGRAPHY

American Diabetes Association consensus statement: Detection and management of lipid disorders in diabetes. *Diabetes Care* 16 (Suppl. 2):106–12, 1993

DCCT Research Group: The effect of intensive treatment of diabetes on the development and progression of long-term complications on insulin-dependent diabetes mellitus. *N Engl J Med* 329:977–86, 1993

Fielding JE: Smoking: health effects and control. *N Engl J Med* 313:491–98, 555–60, 1985

Garg A: Management of dyslipidemia in IDDM patients. *Diabetes Care* 17:224–34, 1994

Kannel WB, MeGee DL: Diabetes and glucose tolerance as risk factors for cardiovascular disease: the Framingham study. *Diabetes Care* 2:120–26, 1979

Lipid Research Clinics Program: The Lipid Research Clinics coronary primary prevention trial results. *JAMA* 251:351–74, 1984

Suarez L, Barrett-Connor E: Interaction between cigarette smoking and diabetes mellitus in the prediction of death attributed to cardiovascular disease. *Am J Epidemiol* 120:670–75, 1984

Limited Joint Mobility

INTRODUCTION

Limited joint mobility (LJM) is a potentially important clinical marker for diabetes complications such as retinopathy, nephropathy, neuropathy, statural growth abnormalities, hypertension, and hepatomegaly. Glycation of tissue proteins associated with chronic hyperglycemia may be responsible for many long-term complications, including LJM.

DETECTION AND EVALUATION

LJM may occur in children or adults, is painless, and causes little disability. Thus, it is unlikely to be brought to the attention of family members or health professionals. The only way to detect LJM is to examine hands and joints as part of routine physical examinations.

To evaluate for LJM, the following should be included. Observe and shake both hands of the patient, noting any sclerodermalike stiffness of the skin. The patient should then be asked to place the hands in a clapping or "prayer" position with forearms as parallel to the floor as possible (Figure 6.10). Any inability to oppose the joints of the fingers and any limitation of flexion or extension of wrist, elbow, neck, or spine should be documented.

If pain or neuromuscular findings (e.g., atrophy, paresthesia) are present, other disorders such as tenosynovitis or carpal tunnel syndrome should be considered. In adults, another possibility is Dupuytren's contracture, which is painless and characterized by palmar nodules and involvement of the 3rd and 4th fingers.

Because there is a relationship between the severity of LJM and the microvascular complications of diabetes, patients found to have LJM at an office visit should be carefully examined for clinical evidence of retinopathy via ophthalmoscopy; for nephropathy by a quantitative determination of urinary microalbumin excretion; and for hypertension, hepatomegaly, and neuropathy by careful clinical examination.

CONCLUSION

Until intervention in the primary glycation process becomes possible or better treatment strategies are perfected, patients with LJM should be periodically assessed for complications and should strive for the best possible glycemic control.

BIBLIOGRAPHY

Brink SJ: *Pediatric and Adolescent Diabetes Mellitus.* Chicago, IL, Year Book, 1987

Rosenbloom AL: Skeletal and joint manifestations of childhood diabetes. *Pediatr Clin N Am* 31: 569–90, 1984

Figure 6.10. Limited Joint Mobility of Increasing Severity

A: normal joint mobility. *B*: bilateral contracture of 5th fingers. *C*: bilaterial contracture of more than 5th fingers. *D*: bilateral wrist involvement.

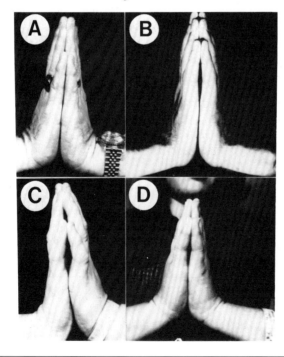

Growth

INTRODUCTION

Abnormalities of height (absolute short stature as well as decreased growth velocity) are known consequences of insulin deficiency. Although the classic example occurs in the extreme and relatively rare Mauriac syndrome (diabetic dwarfism), subtle abnormalities of growth and development are not uncommon among youngsters with type I diabetes. Patients with poorly controlled diabetes have decreased insulin growth factor 1 levels and paradoxical increments in growth hormone levels during the night and in response to provocative stimuli. These abnormalities can be prevented or corrected with better glycemic control.

MAURIAC SYNDROME

Children with Mauriac syndrome are markedly delayed in linear growth and sexual maturation. They are usually pale, appear chronically ill, and have generalized puffiness of the face and extremities and a protuberant abdomen. LJM and hepatomegaly are often present, and laboratory analysis includes not only hyperglycemia and elevated glycohemoglobin levels but also hyperlipidemia.

SUBTLE GROWTH ABNORMALITIES

Less marked growth abnormalities become apparent when large patient populations are studied and subtle growth changes are sought, including a lag in height or weight or a deviation from previously established growth curves (Figures 6.11 and 6.12). Defined in this fashion, 5–10% of youngsters with type I diabetes will not grow well. Children most likely to be affected are those with the earliest onset of diabetes and those who have the worst day-to-day glycemic control and the highest glycohemoglobin levels. Boys are two or three times more likely to have a growth abnormality than girls.

DETERMINING GROWTH RATE

The only way to determine whether growth is adequate is to measure height and weight at each office visit and to plot data on standardized growth charts. Ideally, data should be recorded at least every 3–4 mo; at minimum, height and weight should be measured and recorded annually. Growth data obtained from other family members may be extremely valuable in placing an individual youngster's growth in perspective. Bone-age determination (single radiograph of left wrist and hand compared with standard radiographs) coupled with other hormonal measurements may help assess the need for further evaluation. If growth abnormalities are found, metabolic status should be carefully evaluated and appropriate recommendation for

Figure 6.11. Inadequate Diabetes Control and Growth Abnormalities

Growth deceleration solely from uncontrolled diabetes mellitus. Patient refused to take 2 shots of insulin each day. Most of the time, patient omitted morning insulin and refused to follow any type of meal plan. The family refused psychiatric consultation.
Adapted from Brink SJ: see Bibliography.

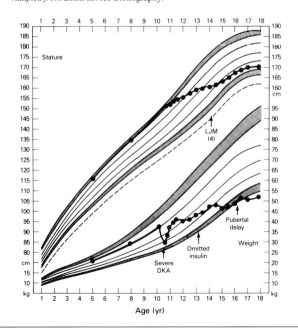

Figure 6.12. Catch-Up Growth Phenomenon With Adequate Insulin

Growth data from child with type I diabetes treated with 1 shot of morning insulin, showing growth deceleration and catch-up growth phenomenon after twice-daily insulin was started.

Adapted from Brink SJ: see Bibliography.

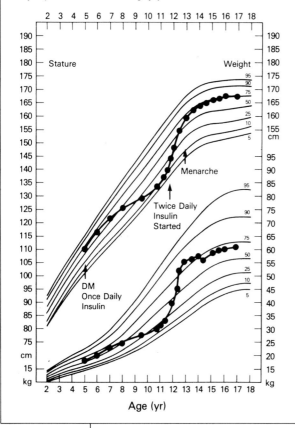

Age (yr)

improvement made, such as changing to an intensified insulin treatment program.

CONCLUSION

Although mild growth retardation may not be totally preventable, evidence strongly indicates that major alterations in growth rate can be avoided by better blood glucose control. Therefore, the definition of adequate diabetes control must include the attainment and maintenance of normal growth and development.

BIBLIOGRAPHY

Brink SJ: *Pediatric and Adolescent Diabetes Mellitus.* Chicago, IL, Year Book, 1987

Clarke WL, Vance ML, Rogol AD: Growth and the child with diabetes mellitus. *Diabetes Care* 16 (Suppl. 3):101–106, 1993

Jackson RL, Guthrie RA: *The Physiological Management of Diabetes in Children.* New York, Medical Examination Publishing, 1986

Travis LB, Brouhard BJ, Schreiner BK: *Diabetes Mellitus in Children and Adolescence.* Philadelphia, PA, Saunders, 1987, p. 206–10

Index

Index

About the American Diabetes Association

The mission of the American Diabetes Association is to prevent and cure diabetes and to improve the lives of all people affected by diabetes.

The American Diabetes Association (ADA) is the nation's leading voluntary health organization dedicated to diabetes research, information, and advocacy. Through the efforts of state affiliates, local chapters, and thousands of volunteers in more than 800 communities across the United States, ADA carries out this mission, educating and building public awareness about diabetes.

As a member of ADA's Professional Section, you access an important network of 11,000 professionals involved in all aspects of diabetes health care — from diabetes treatment and education to diabetes research.

ADA provides a wide range of services and benefits to its professional members, including discounted registration fees for scientific meetings and education programs at the local and national levels; a subscription to one of ADA's professional journals; discounts on the entire library of ADA journals and books; listing in the *Professional Section Membership Directory*; council membership; a free subscription to *Professional Section News*, ADA's quarterly member newsletter; and the latest *Clinical Practice Recommendations*, a publication of ADA's official policies on standards of diabetes treatment and patient education.

For more information about membership, contact:

American Diabetes Association
Customer Service Department
1660 Duke Street
Alexandria, VA 22314
(800) 232-3472 or (703) 549-1500

American Diabetes Association's Prestigious Research Journals

DIABETES
The world's most cited journal in the field devoted to basic diabetes research. Contains major scientific papers related to the molecular, biochemical, and cellular aspects of diabetes. 12 issues/yr.

Professional members: $50, US/Mex ($53.50, Canadian residents, includes GST)
$105 International

Nonmembers: $100, US/Mex ($107, Canadian residents, includes GST)
$155, International

DIABETES CARE
The best-read monthly diabetes clinical research journal. Presents research advances and articles on the latest clinical findings that relate to diagnosis, diet, exercise, monitoring, drug therapy, and complications and their management. Includes analysis and comment on what the latest findings mean for you and your patients. 12 issues/yr.

Professional members: $50, US/Mex ($53.50, Canadian residents, includes GST)
$105, International

Nonmembers: $75, US/Mex ($80.25, Canadian residents, includes GST)
$130, International

DIABETES REVIEWS
World-renowned diabetes investigators review specific topics in their fields and discuss the clinical significance of their own research. Each issue is devoted to a single topic and explores the hottest issues in the field in concise, review format. 4 issues/yr.

Professional members: $45, US/Mex ($48.15, Canadian residents, includes GST)
$65, International

Nonmembers: $65, US/Mex ($69.55, Canadian residents, includes GST)
$85, International

CLINICAL DIABETES
Newsletter geared toward professional with busy schedules. Presents in-depth reviews on important topics in diabetes treatment, plus medical and legal case studies and digests of current research. 6 issues/yr.

Professional members: $15, US/Mex ($16.05, Canadian residents, includes GST)
$21, International

Nonmembers: $20, US/Mex ($21.14, Canadian residents, includes GST)
$26, International

DIABETES SPECTRUM

Concise, ready-to-use resource for diabetes educators and counselors that supports you in counseling patients with diabetes. Translates the latest clinical findings into practical strategies, techniques, and materials you can use immediately to help your patients. 6 issues/yr.

Professional members: $15, US/Mex ($16.05, Canadian residents, includes GST)
$30, International

Nonmembers: $30, US/Mex ($32.10, Canadian residents, includes GST)
$45, International

For more information about subscriptions or if you would like to find out more about **Professional Section Membership**, please call our Customer Service Department at (800) 232-3472 or (703) 549-1500.

Additional Resources From the Clinical Education Series

NEW!

Medical Management of Non-Insulin-Dependent (Type II) Diabetes
formerly: Physician's Guide to Non-Insulin-Dependent (Type II) Diabetes

Thousands have come to rely on the *Physician's Guide* for diagnosing and treating type II diabetes and now the best just got better! This long-awaited revision provides critical information for front-line health professionals and diabetes specialists alike. Completely revised and updated, it features:

- Revised Diagnosis and Classification Criteria
- Updated Information on Pathogenesis
- New Strategies for Achieving Better Metabolic Control
- New Information on Preventing and Treating Diabetes Complications

This book will help you translate the lastest advances in diabetes management into superior patient care. And its succinct, readable format and thorough index make it easy to find the information you need in seconds! 1994. Softcover. #PMMT2
Nonmember: $37.50; Member: $29.95

NEW!

Therapy for Diabetes Mellitus and Related Disorders, 2nd Edition

Put the knowledge of more than 50 diabetes experts right at your fingertips! Updated to reflect DCCT findings and new treatment recommendations, each chapter focuses on a different aspect of diabetes and its complications, presenting a concise, practical approach to treatment. Contains cutting edge treatment information, including: the latest drug therapies; treating diabetic nerve, eye, and kidney disorders; psychosocial issues; managing ketoacidosis and hyperglycemic hyperosmolar coma; cardiovascular complications; and much more! 1994. Softcover. #PMTDRD2
Nonmember: $34.50; Member: $27.50

Medical Management of Pregnancy Complicated by Diabetes

A must-read for anyone involved in treating women with type I, type II, or gestational diabetes! This concise, yet comprehensive guide takes you through every aspect of pregnancy and diabetes, from prepregnancy counseling to postpartum follow-up and everything in between. Provides precise protocols for treatment of both preexisting and gestational diabetes. Tabbed and well indexed for easy access to important information. 1993. Softcover; 136 pages. #PMMPCD
Nonmember: $37.50; Member: $29.95

Cardiovascular Risk Factor Management: A Lecture Program

This 3-hour program focuses on diabetes and its complications as risk factors for atherosclerotic vascular disease. Covers epidemiology, pathophysiology, assessment,

and treatment for each risk factor. Includes case-study discussion and presenter's script. 1993. 92 color slides. #PMCEP3SS
Nonmember: $250.00; Member: $200.00

Managing Diabetes in the '90s: A Lecture Program

Developed to give students a basic overview of diabetes, this color slide program discusses the screening, diagnosis, and management of type I, type II, and gestational diabetes mellitus. The accompanying presenter's script includes case studies and a hard copy of each slide. 83 slides. #PMCEPSS
Nonmember: $95.00; Member: $75.00

Nutrition Guide for Professionals: Diabetes Education and Meal Planning

This publication helps you effectively use the *Exchange Lists for Meal Planning* to create individualized meal plans for your patients. This book is vital to helping you understand the critical role nutrition plays in diabetes management. It also expands on the meal-planning model to include alternatives to the exchange system. Softcover. #PNNG
Nonmember: $12.95; Member: $11.00

Diabetic Foot Care

Prepared by the ADA Council on Foot Care, this booklet contains important information about preventing and treating serious foot problems caused by diabetes. Left unchecked, these problems frequently lead to amputations—something you and your patients both want to avoid if possible. Emphasizes educating patients about proper foot care and routine evaluations to catch problems before they progress. Softcover. #PMFOOT
Nonmember: $5.75; Member: $4.50

Order These Valuable Publications Today!

Yes! Please send me:

		Qty.	Price	Total
Medical Management of Type I Diabetes	#PMMT1_____		@$_____each	= $_____
Medical Management of Type II Diabetes	#PMMT2_____		@$_____each	= $_____
Therapy for Diabetes Mellitus, 2nd Edition	#PMTDRD2_____		@$_____each	= $_____
Medical Management of Pregnancy Complicated by Diabetes	#PMMPCD_____		@$_____each	= $_____
Cardiovascular Risk Factor Management	#PMCEP3SS_____		@$_____each	= $_____
Managing Diabetes in the '90s	#PMCEPSS_____		@$_____each	= $_____
Nutrition Guide for Professionals	#PNNG_____		@$_____each	= $_____
Diabetic Foot Care	#PMFOOT_____		@$_____each	= $_____

Publications Subtotal: $_____

VA Residents Add 4.5% Sales Tax: $_____

Shipping & Handling (based on subtotal): $_____

Grand Total: $_____

Allow 2–3 weeks for shipment. Add $3.00 to shipping & handling for each additional shipping address. Add $15 to shipping & handling for each international shipment. Foreign orders must be paid in U.S. funds, drawn on a U.S. bank. Prices subject to change without notice.

Name_____

Address_____

City/State/Zip_____

Payment enclosed (check or money order) OR

Charge my: ❏ VISA   ❏ MC   ❏ AMEX

Account #_____

Signature_____ Exp. Date_____

Shipping & Handling Chart
up to $30.00 . . . . . .add $3.00
$30.01–$50.00 . . .add $4.00
over $50.00 . . . . . .add 8% of order

Mail to:

American Diabetes Association
1970 Chain Bridge Road
McLean, VA 22109-0592

PH79401

Order These Valuable Publications Today!

Yes! Please send me:

		Qty.	Price	Total
Medical Management of Type I Diabetes	#PMMT1_____		@$_____	each = $_____
Medical Management of Type II Diabetes	#PMMT2_____		@$_____	each = $_____
Therapy for Diabetes Mellitus, 2nd Edition	#PMTDRD2_____		@$_____	each = $_____
Medical Management of Pregnancy Complicated by Diabetes	#PMMPCD_____		@$_____	each = $_____
Cardiovascular Risk Factor Management	#PMCEP3SS_____		@$_____	each = $_____
Managing Diabetes in the '90s	#PMCEPSS_____		@$_____	each = $_____
Nutrition Guide for Professionals	#PNNG_____		@$_____	each = $_____
Diabetic Foot Care	#PMFOOT_____		@$_____	each = $_____

Publications Subtotal: $_____

VA Residents Add 4.5% Sales Tax: $_____

Shipping & Handling (based on subtotal): $_____

Grand Total: $_____

Allow 2–3 weeks for shipment. Add $3.00 to shipping & handling for each additional shipping address. Add $15 to shipping & handling for each international shipment. Foreign orders must be paid in U.S. funds, drawn on a U.S. bank. Prices subject to change without notice.

Name_____

Address_____

City/State/Zip_____

Payment enclosed (check or money order) OR

Charge my: ❑ VISA ❑ MC ❑ AMEX

Account #_____

Signature_____ Exp. Date_____

Shipping & Handling Chart
up to $30.00 . . . . . .add $3.00
$30.01–$50.00 . . .add $4.00
over $50.00 . . . . . .add 8% of order

Mail to:

American Diabetes Association
1970 Chain Bridge Road
McLean, VA 22109-0592

PH79401